Motor neurone disease

Motor neurone disease is one of the most difficult diseases to manage medically and socially. A disease which leads to the loss of most muscle systems of the body, it has no known cause and no cure. For this reason, clinicians have traditionally been reluctant to reveal the diagnosis to sufferers or their families, and the condition had become known as one of the best kept secrets of medical practice. However, in recent years a number of organisations have been set up to support people who have the condition and their families, and, consequently, the public profile of the condition has changed dramatically.

Motor Neurone Disease provides an extremely helpful guide to the medical facts relating to the condition and considers the psychosocial effects on sufferers and those who care for them. It demonstrates how sufferers constantly have to adapt to their increasing loss of muscular ability and how they manage their lives accordingly. It is essential reading for doctors, nurses, social workers and therapists, as well as people who have the condition, their families and carers.

Ian Robinson is Director of The John Bevan MND Research Unit and is a Senior Lecturer in Human Sciences at Brunel University. **Maggie Hunter** is a Lecturer and Research Fellow in Human Sciences at Brunel University.

The Experience of Illness
Series editors: Ray Fitzpatrick and Stanton Newman

Motor Neurone Disease

This b~ ~

Ian Robinson and Maggie Hunter

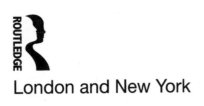

London and New York

First published 1998
by Routledge
11 New Fetter Lane, London EC4P 4EE

Simultaneously published in the USA and Canada
by Routledge
29 West 35th Street, New York, NY 10001

Typeset in Times by Routledge
Printed and bound in Great Britain by Creative Print and
Design (Wales), Ebbw Vale

British Library Cataloguing in Publication Data
A catalogue record for this book is available from the British
Library

Library of Congress Cataloging in Publication Data
Robinson, Ian, 1943–
Motor neurone disease / Ian Robinson and Maggie Hunter.
p. cm. – (Experience of illness)
Includes bibliographical references and index.
1. Amyotrophic lateral sclerosis. I. Hunter, Maggie, 1948–
II. Title. III. Series.
RC406.A24R62   1998
616.8'3–dc21   97–32221
                                                                          CIP

ISBN 0–415–09711–8

Contents

Series Editor's preface

Motor neurone disease (MND) refers to a range of disorders that impact on the nervous system and its control of muscles. The poor prognosis that commonly is associated with the disease means that individuals experience MND as a series of major challenges to the self and to the body. The diagnosis is an acute shock to the individual, but the meaning of the diagnosis is something that is continually discovered.

Ian Robinson is a senior and experienced social scientist who has researched and written widely on the impact of neurological disorders. An earlier volume in this series sensitively and authoritatively discussed the hopes, frustrations and dilemmas of individuals with multiple sclerosis. Here he and his colleague Maggie Hunter, a psychologist with longstanding research interests in neurological diseases, draw on their extensive research with individuals experiencing motor neurone disease to provide a graphic account of the disorder from the perspective of the individual and his or her carers.

Robinson and Hunter emphasise that now is a crucial time for all concerned with MND. There are, for the first time, drugs available that, it is hoped, may have an effect on the course of the disease. Increasingly imaginative and constructive technology is being developed to reduce the handicap of the disorder. Information is itself a vital resource that can aid the individual in finding solutions to challenges and hazards of the disease. Robinson and Hunter find a realistic balance in their analysis of the situation of individuals with MND. On the one hand they describe the physical limitations and problems that increasingly follow onset. On the other, theirs is a humane and encouraging account of individuals', carers' and the health service's search for solutions. This volume is essential for anyone wanting to gain insight into the experience of MND.

Ray Fitzpatrick, 1997

Preface

This book has been long in the writing. It is based on many years of research with people with motor neurone disease (MND) and their families, and specifically originated from a large research project on the disease established at Brunel University, West London, through the initiative of the late John Bevan and his family, friends and colleagues, with the support of the Motor Neurone Disease Association. The charity which John Bevan and others established – Monitor – was set up to support this research, and to provide additional therapy for people with MND. We are particularly grateful to Judith Harte, Director of Monitor; Lynne Brooke, Chairman of the Charity, as well as the other Trustees – most notably Neil Hughes and Frank Clifford Rose, for their continuing and warm support for our research on MND, which has been undertaken in the John Bevan MND Research Unit.

We are especially grateful to Ray Fitzpatrick, and to Heather Gibson of Routledge, for their considerable tolerance and good humour in the face of the lengthy delays in the production of the book. In addition Ian Robinson would particularly like to acknowledge the sacrifices made by his family during a lengthy summer which at every point was accompanied by the considerable commitment required to complete the text.

The book has been written primarily within a qualitative methodological framework, complementing other significant quantitative work produced in the John Bevan MND Unit, most notably by Stuart Neilson, whose strikingly original epidemiological research on MND has very profitably redirected some previously rather sterile and circular debates on the environmental origins of the disease. In addition Stuart Neilson has been instrumental in setting up and maintaining the overall data resources of the John Bevan MND

Research Unit, and particularly in the context of this work continues to oversee and develop the Unit's international electronic sources of information for people with MND and their relatives, as well as for the scientific community. We are particularly grateful to him for his skills and support in providing material for this book.

The book itself draws on a number of key sources of information, apart from relevant, and widely available, scientific and social scientific literature. These sources include: international data, especially mortality data on the disease; the life stories of over three hundred people with MND and their relatives, written to assist the work of the John Bevan MND Research Unit; questionnaire-based surveys undertaken by the Unit of a large cohort of people with the disease and their relatives; the rapidly increasing electronic resource of the international Amyotrophic Lateral Sclerosis Interest Group (ALSIG) weekly Newsletter, and through that Newsletter, information from other electronic data resources on MND; literature produced by voluntary organisations including the Motor Neurone Disease Association (MNDA) in Britain, and the ALSA (Amyotrophic Lateral Sclerosis Association) in the United States, and other equivalent organisations throughout the world; and finally many and lengthy interviews and discussions with people with MND, their relatives, and many professional staff concerned with their health care. All names, and other identifying information, have been changed in the accounts to preserve the anonymity of those contributing to this book.

We have come into contact with many extraordinary people during the course of this work, who both directly and indirectly have made an invaluable contribution to our research on MND. We thank them all for their interest and for their forbearance in the midst of far more important issues to which they have had to attend, for without their personal interest and enthusiasm we truly could not have written this book. Alas, many of those with MND whom we knew well have now died, but we hope that their families and friends, and others who currently have the condition will find that we have reflected some of their experiences of living and dying with the disease with accuracy and sensitivity. We must say, however, to those who read this book, that experiencing and managing MND is a difficult process for everyone involved, and we have not shied away from documenting all of those difficulties which touch every facet of how people with the disease live and die.

Chapter 1

Understanding motor neurone disease
The medical context

Until very recently motor neurone disease (MND) was known amongst the community of those whom it touched as a 'hidden secret'. Not only did the diagnosis of the disease often appear to be hidden from the patient and frequently from their family, it was a condition which many of those concerned with medical care were reluctant to acknowledge openly for the issues involved in managing people diagnosed with the disease were – and still are – deemed to be profoundly demanding and difficult. Of all diseases, until recently, it has appeared to be the one which has most highlighted medical impotence in relation to even the possibility of a cure, as well as revealing the paucity of weapons in the armoury of those managing the care of people affected by the condition.

However the public profile of motor neurone disease has been raised considerably in recent years. In this process the role of particular celebrated individuals with the disease has been exceptionally important. The late actor David Niven, who died from the disease, gave MND transatlantic prominence. Other leading figures in Britain who also died from the disease were the former England football (soccer) manager Don Revie, and the former Director General of the BBC, Ian Trethowan; whilst in the United States a key senator, Jacob Javits, also succumbed to MND. However, perhaps the two most widely known figures who have had the condition are Stephen Hawking, the celebrated physicist, who – at the time of writing – is still alive, and in the United States, in particular the late Lou Gehrig, one of the most famous men in baseball history, after whom MND has become almost universally and colloquially known in North America – that is, as 'Lou Gehrig's disease'. In many ways this small number of public figures epitomise key features of the disease, both in its demographic and symptomatic characteristics, and in the tragedy that the disease is often considered to represent.

David Niven, Don Revie, Ian Trethowan and Jacob Javits were all men in late middle age, that is in their late fifties or sixties, which is by far the most common time of life when the disease appears to strike. These four men are, in a sense, proxies for the many others, predominantly men, in whom MND is expressed at or about the time of usual retirement from paid employment in the industrialised world. There is no known causal link between the disease and the psychological or social aspects of the retirement process itself, but the coincidence of the two leads to an added set of difficulties with the onset of MND. The personal poignancy of these men's encounters with MND lies in the ways in which their earlier robust and energetic lives were rapidly reduced in degree and kind as their physical capacities shrank through the trepidations of the disease, which led to major bodily limitations occurring before their perceived 'rightful time' in late old age.

Stephen Hawking and Lou Gehrig, who were both well under forty when the first symptoms of the disease appeared, have been demographic exceptions to the most usual age ranges in which MND occurs. However the relatively atypical incidence of the disease in those under forty has, for profound social and other reasons, given their plight a significance way beyond that which might be statistically warranted. Lou Gehrig, for example, who played his baseball for the New York Yankees was called the 'Ironman', and had rewritten the baseball record books with his prodigious feats. At the peak of his career at the age of thirty-six he was diagnosed with the disease, and died two years later. Thereafter his name, following his public struggle with the onset and progress of MND, entered everyday North American vocabulary. The stark contrast between his former physical prowess and his rapid bodily decline to death at such a young age epitomises, for many – and not only in North America – the intractable, and socially as well as physically, pernicious nature of the disease.

Stephen Hawking, who has had MND for over twenty years and who is currently in his late forties, by his presence and activities has been instrumental in demonstrating the dramatic effects of the disease to a global audience. He has little conventional muscular control, is now confined to a wheelchair, and uses a voice synthesiser as his main means of public communication. He has gained many international honours for his work on the origins of the universe. He has also become a strikingly visible and literal embodiment of the major physical effects of the disease, on the one hand, and, on the other, of the apparently dramatic possibilities through which the inner and less visible resources of the (super)human mind and a determined personal will can rise above and beyond the physically damaged body. Indeed, for many, the unfathomable paradox of Stephen Hawking's life with MND is seen in the almost limitless universe he majestically surveys, set against the fragility and frailty of his physical form. In more general terms, this paradox provides a common way of understanding and describing the progressive effects of MND – as an individual (a mind) imprisoned within an increasingly unusable body. In addition, the most salient aspect of Stephen Hawking's situation for many people with MND is that he is still alive so long after the onset of the disease, and the inference is drawn by such people that it is his mind, his 'brain power', that has led to his extraordinarily long life with the disease, when almost all others with the condition would have died.

However, given the multiplicity of diseases which affect many people at all stages of their lives, and which themselves produce suffering in no small measure, these images of motor neurone disease as producing a unique set of social and personal, as well as medical consequences deserve special scrutiny. This book is therefore essentially an exploration of the basis and extent to which MND might be considered as an extraordinary and telling disease which stands apart from almost all others, in the manner of its appearance, its course, its effects on those who are diagnosed with it and its mode of management by them and others.

THE NATURE OF MOTOR NEURONE DISEASE

Motor neurone diseases can be considered to be a family of conditions all centred on the destruction in various ways, at various ages, and with various effects of motor neurones. Motor neurones are effectively electrical junction boxes occurring in all parts of the human nervous system. They are a vital link throughout the nervous system in managing the transmission of electrical messages from the brain which control all muscular activity. Even though the normal ageing process leads to the loss of some motor neurones and a decline in the efficiency of others, considerable redundancy in their provision means many such neurones can malfunction in the ageing process and still leave no major loss in muscular control.

However, in the motor neurone diseases, massive damage to motor neurones at various sites in the nervous system gradually leads to a loss of muscular control which increasingly becomes evident to those affected by these conditions.

It is almost certain that by the time the loss of muscular control becomes evident, the damage sustained to the motor neurones will already have been substantial. As many of the motor neurone diseases – although not all – occur relatively late in life, it is likely that damage has been increasingly occurring over many years, and even possibly many decades, before symptoms are made manifest to individuals. When those symptoms are evident, muscles are already gradually weakening, leading in the end to their wasting or atrophy. This process, in the most commonly occurring forms of the disease, is almost always rapidly progressive with a fatal outcome for the individual, usually through respiratory complications when the disease is very advanced.

In investigating motor neurone disease and its effects, it is important to be aware at the outset of terminological differences. There are distinct terms in different countries which confusingly appear to apply to the same condition and which reflect different clinical and scientific traditions. For clinicians and scientists in North America and many other countries, 'motor neurone disease' is often employed as a generic category applying to all the many diseases and conditions associated with damage to the motor neurones. In Britain, and in a number of European countries, 'motor neurone disease' is a term usually applied to a specific form of that damage and its consequences. Furthermore, the particular disease usually referred to as 'motor neurone disease' (MND) in Britain, is often called by the more complex term 'amyotrophic lateral sclerosis' (ALS) in North America, or, as has been noted, Lou Gehrig's disease. In fact the respective European and North American terms (MND and ALS) cover by far the vast majority (well over 90 per cent) of all cases of the motor neurone diseases (Tandon and Bradley 1985), and are considered as referring to what is sometimes described as the 'classic' form of the disease. However, just to compound the terminological problems, the classic form of the disease is often known in France and French-speaking countries, as 'le maladie de Charcot', after Charcot the famous nineteenth-century French neurologist who is attributed with first identifying and cataloguing the effects of the condition (Charcot 1874).

Whilst motor neurone disease (MND) is perhaps a more self-evident term for the condition, the term Amyotrophic Lateral Sclerosis (ALS) is derived from a different source. 'A-myo-trophic' is a term of Greek derivation. In this context 'a' means no or negative, 'myo' refers to muscle, and 'trophic' means nourishment, thus: 'no muscle nourishment or nutrition'. When a muscle has no nutrition, it 'atrophies' or wastes away. 'Lateral' identifies the areas where the nerve cells that transmit messages (or provide 'nutrition') to the muscles are located. As this area degenerates, it leads to scarring or hardening – 'sclerosis' – in the region where the damage has occurred.

In lay terms, the terminological differences have led to some confusion in the transferability of information from North America, and elsewhere in the world, to Britain. In interpreting both information for those with the disease and the increasingly voluminous scientific and medical literature, considerable care is needed to clarify whether the generic and all embracing category 'motor neurone diseases' is the focus, or the particular and individual disease category 'motor neurone disease' (MND/ALS) – which is the focus of this account. Scientists and clinicians, being essentially engaged in a continuous process of taxonomising diseases, have been able to circumnavigate these complexities with greater ease, although there are still occasional difficulties in the process of communication. This particular account is centred on the disease MND/ALS, which will now be the term employed here and which, with its various sub-categories, is the disease most frequently the object of discussion and analysis, both in the public domain and scientifically and medically.

THE CLASSIFICATION, DIAGNOSIS AND SYMPTOMS OF MND/ALS

MND/ALS, and associated conditions, may affect all or some motor neurones. In particular, three general sites in the nervous system are often used as a basis on which different clinical types of the diseases are distinguished by virtue of the inferences drawn from the symptoms initially presented by people with the disease. These three sites are in the upper motor neurones occurring in the brain and upper part of the spinal cord; in the lower motor neurones occurring in the lower parts of the spinal cord and nervous system, and in the motor neurones in the brain stem or bulbar area. These sites may be affected individually or in combination, either simultaneously or consecutively, but it is likely that as the disease advances more and more sites will be explicitly involved, made evident through the increasing range and severity of symptoms.

However standard classifications of the motor neurone diseases – using the term in a generic sense – are based not only on the clinical similarities and differences between them, but also on their assumed origins, possible causes and, in certain cases, their geographical location. Debates over classification have been particularly important in clinical research on both causes and possible approaches to the management of the disease. A great deal of scientific and clinical endeavour has been devoted to attempting to establish typical and discrete categories of the disease, not only on the basis of distinctive sets of pathologies, but particularly on their rates of progression, outcomes and possible symptomatic management. From the point of view of a person with MND/ALS, such classificatory information is also vital, as we shall discuss in later chapters, for with a prognosis that is generally so poor, any – even slightly – less virulent form of the disease is a modestly welcome development. As with all diseases, there are both relatively standard classifications and some debate over the exact relationship between sub-categories within them. Mitsumoto and Norris's (1994) classification of the major forms of motor neurone disease is sufficiently clear and widely used to form the basis of this analysis. The taxonomy is as follows:

(a) *Sporadic MND/ALS*

This form of the disease, which comprises 90–95 per cent of all cases, is distinguished by the absence of any known family history of the condition. It is often further sub-divided for clinical purposes into:

- *Classical MND/ALS*: the particular form of the disease identified by Charcot involving motor neurones in many parts of the upper and lower nervous system – about two-thirds of all sporadic cases.
- *Progressive Bulbar Palsy*: a form of the disease initially affecting the brainstem (bulbar) area and clinically affecting speech and swallowing in the early stages (approximately 25 per cent of sporadic cases begin in this form).
- *Progressive Muscular Atrophy*: this form of the disease primarily relates to damage initially to motor neurones in the lower nervous system, and comprises about 10 per cent of all

sporadic cases, but may progress to involve the upper motor neurones.

- *Primary Lateral Sclerosis*: a rarer form of the disease in which only the upper motor neurones are involved.

It is not clear whether these sporadic forms of the disease are completely distinguishable, for although initial presentation may appear to be of one form rather than another, as we have noted, in many cases motor neurones in all parts of the nervous system become progressively involved. In such cases highly focused clinical symptoms at first develop into an increasingly all-embracing loss of muscle function.

(b) *Familial MND/ALS*

Traditionally familial forms of the disease occur in approximately 5–10 per cent of all cases, where more than one member of the same family is known to have been diagnosed with the disease, either in the same or consecutive generations. However, there is little clinical difference between the symptoms and course of the familial and sporadic forms of the disease, although autopsy examinations suggest a slightly different pathology.

(c) *Other forms of MND/ALS*

A number of other forms of MND/ALS have been identified which are relatively rare and/or highly geographically localised. *Western Pacific MND/ALS* is found on the island of Guam, and in two other local areas in the Pacific Region. This disease was characterised by a very high local prevalence, but in recent years there has been a very rapid local decline, which has led to considerable investigation of environmental and related causes. *Juvenile MND/ALS* is very rare, but may occur occasionally in those between twelve and sixteen, and its cause and relationship to sporadic MND/ALS is not clear. Finally there are a wide range of very rare *MND/ALS type diseases with definable causes* associated with some other conditions (such as poliomyelitis), or with certain kinds of neurotoxicity (such as that from lead or mercury).

It is often indicated by neurologists that although there is still no definitive laboratory test for MND/ALS, its clinical identification is, in the context of other neurological conditions, relatively clear (Bradley 1994). Such identification is usually made by observing and examining the particular ways in which muscle control, action and tone are currently affected by the disease, and the clinical history which has led to current signs and symptoms. Diagnosis is, in effect, by exclusion, through the elimination of other conditions which might be associated with apparent motor neurone disease-like symptoms, and through the confirmation of the formal clinical expression of motor neurone damage or destruction. In principle, there are an exhaustive and continuing range of tests which can be conducted to investigate many other very rare, and possible – though improbable – causes of the symptoms. In most cases, however, what Bradley describes as 'the investigation of time' (1994: 23) is sufficient to reveal the identity of the disease, for a combination of a distinctive clinical profile and the inexorable progression in key neurological symptoms is likely itself to provide conclusive evidence of its existence. Given the implications of a categorical diagnosis of MND/ALS, many clinicians appear to be particularly cautious in acting on their initial – for the most part correct – judgements about the usually distinctive symptomatic patterns of the disease.

MND/ALS affecting the upper motor neurones is often characterised clinically by symptoms such as spasticity (continued contractions in particular muscles), hyperreflexia (exaggerated reflexes in muscle groups), and an almost unique situation in MND/ALS where, as Mitsumoto describes, 'severely wasted, nearly paralysed muscles have brisk reflexes' (1994: 8). Lower motor neurone signs of the disease may include a combination of substantial muscle weakness, in addition to loss of coordination and movement, particular weakness in neck muscles controlling head position and movement, muscle wasting or atrophy, fasciculations – rapid and fine involuntary muscle movements ('twitches'), and a loss of muscle tone and cramps. Brainstem (bulbar) damage to motor neurones may result in a range of difficulties with speech (dysarthria) based on increasing problems with the relevant complex muscular control. At an advanced stage, speech may be impossible (anarthria). Associated and major difficulties in chewing and swallowing (dysphagia) may also occur with bulbar damage and there may be a problem with 'drooling' as the ability to swallow excess saliva becomes impaired. A range of other symptoms may occur at various stages in the disease including increasingly significant respiratory problems as the muscular control of the diaphragm is affected and as the posture of people with the disease affects their respiration. Often fatigue and substantial weight loss occur, the latter being associated particularly with the decline in muscle mass, and the effects of bulbar symptoms which lead to increasing difficulty in food intake.

This substantial catalogue of symptoms may be present in varying combinations and varying severities, depending on the stage of the disease and the degree to which some or all of the motor neurones are affected. In colloquial and everyday terms, early symptoms of MND/ALS may include initially tripping up, dropping things, abnormal fatigue of the arms and/or legs, slurred speech, and unusual and persistent muscle cramps and twitches. The hands and feet may be affected first, causing difficulty in walking or using the hands for the activities of daily living such as dressing, washing and buttoning clothes.

About 25 per cent of people with MND/ALS find that difficulties or changes in using their voice and swallowing are the first symptoms that they notice. Such people would be most often diagnosed as having progressive bulbar palsy, unless there were a range of other symptoms simultaneously present. However the majority of those with MND/ALS first notice that one or more of their limbs are affected – about 50 per cent notice the onset through difficulties with muscular control of their arms or hands, and about 25 per cent through problems in the muscular control of their legs.

An important caveat to the possible presence of the wide range of symptoms set out in this section is that the senses of sight, touch, hearing, taste and smell are very rarely affected in MND/ALS. Similarly the muscles of the eyes and bladder are generally not impaired by the disease, as are neither sexual function nor drive. The mind and intellectual capacity does not appear to be directly affected by MND/ALS itself. However, given the older ages at which the disease is generally diagnosed, it is likely – as with other older people – that a proportion of those with MND/ALS will have some reduced cognitive capacity, and a much smaller proportion of others will have seriously affected cognitive capacity (dementia). Indeed, one of the personally and socially (as well as medically) difficult issues raised by the disease is self-evidently the relationship between an active mind and a physically diminished body.

As can be extrapolated from this lengthy list of potential symptoms, with advancement of the disease there are likely to be a multiplicity of issues requiring detailed, painstaking and exhaustive management by physicians and other health care professionals, by people with MND/ALS themselves, and perhaps most of all by others – family and friends – involved informally with the person with the disease. As we have described, almost all unassisted muscular activity becomes difficult, and then virtually impossible, affecting not only what in lay terms would be considered to be issues of 'normal' mobility, but often even more fundamental functions. Thus, in formal managerial terms there may be, in addition to the 'usual' problems associated with being wheelchair or bedbound, major difficulties associated with breathing, swallowing (and choking), eating and drinking, and frequently with inter-personal communication.

The precise sequence in which this formidable range of difficulties occur varies from one person to another. In people with early bulbar symptoms, major problems can arise very quickly in relation to swallowing, with its associated difficulties of control of saliva and choking, and voice-based communication. On the other hand, those with lower motor neurone based symptoms may not lose muscular control over such bulbar functions for several years, and indeed some may never do so. However, for most people with MND/ALS, potentially life-threatening debilitation in muscular control of breathing and swallowing will occur at some point in the disease.

THE DEMOGRAPHIC PATTERNS AND DISTRIBUTION OF MND/ALS

We have already implied that MND/ALS is primarily a disease of late middle age. Indeed, the mean ages at which research reports indicate the disease is usually expressed are almost invariably in the late fifties or early sixties. The disease most frequently occurs in the fifth and sixth decades of life, with smaller numbers in the fourth and seventh decades, and there is relatively rarely occurrence outside this range (Williams and Windebank 1991). MND/ALS may thus be considered as primarily a disease associated with ageing, although it tends to be expressed rather earlier than other neurological diseases with different symptomologies, such as Parkinson's disease and Alzheimer's disease, with which epidemiological parallels are sometimes drawn. However the gender distribution of the disease has been one of its particular hallmarks with nearly two-thirds of those with MND/ALS being men (Buckley et al. 1983), although some research has suggested that the gender balance is becoming more equal (Neilson et al. 1993a).

For many years, MND/ALS was considered to be a disease

which was distributed relatively uniformly – with a few very notable exceptions. Indeed, compared to many other neurological conditions, this degree of uniformity – in terms of the incidence of the disease between 0.4 and 2.4 persons annually per 100,000 population – was considered both exceptional and puzzling (Molgaard 1993a). In this respect, the very few areas of the world where the incidence appeared to be substantially greater became the focus of considerable epidemiological interest. The exceptions to the uniform pattern appeared to be most notably the Chamorro population of Guam in the Marianas Islands in the Western Pacific, the Kii peninsula of Japan and a region of Western New Guinea, all of which had an incidence of an MND/ALS syndrome which was far higher than elsewhere. In Guam, for example, the incidence amongst the Chamorro people was 50–100 times greater than the sporadic form of the disease in the United States, with a mean age of onset in the mid-forties rather than the early sixties (Kurland and Radhakrishnan 1993). However, in recent times the incidence of the condition has substantially decreased in Guam, and even more for those Chamorros who migrated from the island (Molgaard 1993b). On the other hand, there have been studies demonstrating a considerable rise in numbers of cases of the disease in industrialised countries especially in older age groups over the last thirty years (Lilienfeld *et al.* 1989), whilst the incidence in developing countries still appears to be relatively low (Olivares *et al.* 1972). These studies have largely redirected research attention back to the industrialised world, and refocused concern on the supposedly uniform distribution of the disease. Debate has centred, on the one hand, on whether the recent growing disparity in the distribution of MND/ALS was an 'artefact' of differential diagnosis and recording – that is neurologists and other physicians were diagnosing more of the *existing* cases which had previously been missed or wrongly diagnosed – or, on the other hand, whether there was a 'real' increase in the incidence of the disease due to some unknown factor.

The conventional view has been that the 'artefact' explanation was the more powerful, especially in the light of the increased public profile of the disease and the corresponding substantial research interest (Swash *et al.* 1989). However, whilst some of the increase in incidence might plausibly be accounted for in this way, the rise has been general and inexorable in countries with completely different health care systems, very different ratios of neurologists and physicians to the at-risk population, very different public debates about the disease and widely varied sizes and roles of national voluntary – patient-based – organisations. Thus, it does appear that the rise is in large measure a 'real' increase in cases of MND/ALS which is leading not only to more cases in the older age groups, but conversely not only a relative but an absolute decline in people with the disease under the age of fifty (Neilson *et al.* 1993a). However, the prevalence of the disease, that is the pool of people who currently have the condition, is – unlike many other medical conditions – growing relatively little in size. This is self-evidently because mortality from the disease is so high that almost as many people are 'lost' to that pool each year through death as are added to it by new cases.

THE CAUSES OF MND/ALS

The cause or causes of most forms of MND/ALS have been a mystery until very recently. However, substantial strides have been made in the last five years in identifying factors, especially genetic factors, which appear to be firmly linked to the genesis of the condition. The precise link between genetic and environmental factors which may operate in triggering the disease or in accelerating its course is, however, still unclear in the majority of cases.

Although it has been known for many decades that there is a familial form of MND/ALS – constituting, as we have noted, 5–10 per cent of all cases – it was thought that the much more frequent sporadic form of the disease was associated with one or more environmental factors of some kind, rather than with genetic factors. Almost by definition, sporadic MND/ALS was deemed to be unlikely to be linked to what, in lay terms, could be described as family or constitutional causes. In this respect, the search for the cause(s) of the disease has both been based on its epidemiology (its distribution and demography) and on detailed laboratory work on its pathology – on the motor neurones themselves, and on what processes might have led inside the body to their destruction. To a large degree these two approaches have meshed together as knowledge about potentially neurotoxic (nervous system damaging) substances – derived from animal research, from studies of other diseases and conditions and from specific attempts to replicate motor neurone destruction – has been considered in the light of the characteristics of people with MND/ALS and with what damaging substances or environments with which they may have had contact.

Not surprisingly, the high incidence of an MND/ALS syndrome in particular localities in the Pacific region ensured that a great deal of scientific effort was devoted to exploring why these so-called 'hot spots' of the disease existed in anticipation that the clues from such studies would reveal the causes of MND/ALS more generally. Indeed, much of the epidemiological – and a considerable proportion of the laboratory-based – literature for twenty-five years was based on causal possibilities linked to the Pacific forms of the disease. A wide range of potential culprits in the form of neurotoxic factors were located and examined, especially those with whom the Pacific populations had had substantial or extended contact – including indigenous food and food plants, candidate minerals in water or other products, building and related materials, and contact with animals and other peoples who might have introduced or enhanced the likelihood of the syndrome. A complication for this search, which appeared at first to be a helpful coincidence, was the high incidence of other neurological conditions – including two syndromes almost identical to Parkinson's and Alzheimer's diseases. These syndromes, unusually, compared to their occurrence in other locations outside the Pacific region, might occur simultaneously in one individual.

It proved difficult to identify environmental aetiological factors which were common to all the Pacific locations, although it appeared that two of the most plausible were the extensive use by local populations of flour made from the nut of the Cycad (an evergreen palm-like plant) which contained potent neurotoxins, or, in Guam, a depleted intake of calcium and magnesium causing toxic levels of uptake of aluminium. Each of these hypotheses has had its ardent body of supporters, although the Cycad hypothesis appears to be the most plausible, both through animal studies which have revealed major neurological symptoms following administration of the neurotoxins present in the plant (cycasin and BMAA), and paradoxically through the continuing subsequent decline in the incidence of neurological disorders as the use of Cycad flour itself rapidly declined (Kurland and Radhakrishnan 1993).

The detailed relevance of these studies for MND/ALS in the rest of the world was never completely clear, except as an indication that potent neurotoxins can produce potent neurological effects. However, the research led to an intensive search for equivalent candidates elsewhere, with a major focus on heavy metals – especially lead and mercury – with known neurotoxic properties. The research also focused on a number of chemical agents, on contacts with diseases known to damage motor neurones, particularly poliomyelitis, and finally, but rather less intensively, on the influence of plant-based neurotoxins. Laboratory work on these possibilities has been supplemented with epidemiological work seeking to ascertain, through the analysis of medical records and retrospective questioning of people with MND/ALS and control subjects with similar backgrounds, the nature and degree of exposure to possible factors. However, such studies of predominantly older people, even run rigorously with the best of intentions, have had difficulty in accurately identifying relevant factors because of differential memory, problems in identifying the degree as well as the existence of exposure to potentially toxic substances, and the complicated interaction in individuals of many possible aetiological factors over many years (Robinson et al. 1991).

This apparent impasse in penetrating the aetiology of the disease has been largely overcome through what now, in retrospect, appears to have been two parallel sets of approaches to MND/ALS. The first of these has been an innovative set of epidemiological analyses undertaken by Neilson and his colleagues (Neilson et al. 1993a), which for the first time demonstrated that the increase in sporadic cases of the disease in industrialised societies was almost entirely explicable by the increase in population life expectancy in those societies. In addition, the profile of deaths over many years from the disease indicated very strongly that sporadic MND/ALS – in addition to familial MND/ALS – was a condition with a genetic component. It appeared from such analyses that there was a relatively consistently sized but small section of the population susceptible to MND/ALS, and that the increase in overall population life expectancy had allowed more of this susceptible population to reach the ages at which the symptoms of the disease were expressed – whereas previously many would have died from other causes before reaching that point (Neilson et al. 1992). This hypothesis has been shown to be statistically applicable to many industrialised countries – to England (Neilson et al. 1992), the United States (Neilson et al. 1993a), Japan (Neilson et al. 1993b), Sweden (Neilson et al. 1994b), Norway (Neilson et al. 1994b), France (Neilson et al. 1994a) and Spain (Neilson et al. 1996a). Conversely, the reason for the relatively low incidence of MND/ALS in many developing countries is that their population life expectancies are generally lower, and thus many in the sub-populations in those countries susceptible to MND/ALS die earlier in life and thus do not reach the age at which they would express the disease. Paradoxically, therefore, susceptible but healthier (longer-lived) populations of industrialised countries have thereby exposed themselves to an additional but late onset disease.

Contemporaneously with Neilson *et al.*'s research, important publications (Siddique *et al.* (1990), and later in more specific detail Rosen *et al.* (1993)) arose from laboratory-based research locating a significant source of the genetic involvement in familial MND/ALS. In familiar MND/ALS it would appear that about 20 per cent of the cases are associated with a defect (mutation) in the gene responsible for the production of an enzyme called copper/zinc superoxide dismutase (Cu/Zn SOD1). This enzyme is involved in scavenging and clearing damaging toxic substances from the nervous system (particularly anti-oxidants). In a way which is still unclear, mutation in this gene, and thus alteration in the enzyme, leads to the production of MND/ALS. This similarly occurs in transgenic mice when the gene is mutated (Gurney *et al.* 1994). Further dedicated research on genetic involvement in sporadic cases is gradually revealing a complex portfolio of genetic sites which together are likely to point to the basis for individual susceptibility to MND/ALS in those cases.

This genetic research links with another broad strand of work on what is known as excitotoxicity, in which substances normally present in the brain and essential in transmitting messages throughout the nervous system reach damagingly high levels of activity in MND/ALS through changes in their quality and quantity (Duggan and Choi 1994). One of these substances in particular – glutamate – has been especially implicated in motor neurone death. At the same time, the discovery of an increasing number of neurotrophic (nerve growth) factors which appear to be missing in people with MND/ALS, or only present in modest amounts, has directed attention to their role in maintaining the functional status of motor neurones. Such neurotrophic factors are known to be essential for the development and growth of the nervous system. A range of other possible causal mechanisms for MND/ALS are also being investigated.

By far the greatest emphasis on causal mechanisms at present is that centred on understanding the genetic basis of susceptibility to MND/ALS; how such susceptibility becomes triggered to result in the disease, and what then precisely occurs in the nervous system to cause the destruction of motor neurones. Although this body of work has come to be accepted by most scientists as revolutionising the research orientation to the disease, the genetics of sporadic MND/ALS are complex. It is still likely that there are indeed environmentally based triggering factors which provoke the onset of the disease at different times, and possibly accelerating factors which hasten the course of the condition. These factors may still operate in general ways, and Neilson et al.'s analysis of the historical patterns of deaths from the disease in Japan and Spain suggests that there are a range of largely unknown factors which may influence (and accelerate) deaths from the disease, even on a national scale. Controversially, they have hypothesised that radiation may be one amongst possibly many other triggering/accelerating factors in MND/ALS, both historically in Japan (Neilson et al. 1993a, 1996b) and Spain (Neilson et al. 1996c), and contemporarily in England (Neilson et al. 1996b). In this respect, the search for environmental factors linked to the onset of MND/ALS is not ended, but has a new focus. However, the parallel search for a cure for the disease has increasingly built on ways in which genetic and related nervous system defects might be corrected, ameliorated or compensated for in some way.

THE PROGNOSIS AND MANAGEMENT OF MND/ALS

The prognosis for the majority of people with MND/ALS is poor. Most series of such people studied have demonstrated that between 50 per cent and 60 per cent will die within three years of their diagnosis, and a further 20 per cent to 30 per cent will not see the end of their fifth year after diagnosis (Mitsumoto 1994). However, some 20 per cent will live beyond five years and 10 per cent reach ten years, and a very few of these will live two or more decades after diagnosis. On the other hand, there are people with the disease who will rapidly deteriorate and die within a few months, but for those still alive four years after the diagnosis their prospects for further survival increase. In general, the poorest prognoses are for those with initial brainstem (bulbar) symptoms as a result of bulbar motor neurone damage, or for those whose symptoms include difficulties with respiration at an early stage. In addition, the older the age at onset the more likely it is that death will occur sooner. As a corollary, the younger the age at onset the more likely it is that people will have a longer life with MND/ALS. Certain forms of MND/ALS also have a better prognosis, particularly primary lateral sclerosis, involving almost entirely upper motor neurones, and progressive muscular atrophy, involving almost entirely lower motor neurones. There is also a form of the disease often described as pseudobulbar palsy in which bulbar symptoms appear to be caused through upper neurone (not bulbar) damage that also has a better prognosis.

Given this substantial range of forms of MND/ALS there is often great difficulty, as well as a considerable reluctance, to estimate survival times for people who are diagnosed with the disease, and very occasionally the disease can appear to stop progressing and become stable for long periods of time – which Norris refers to as the disease 'burning itself out' (1994). Individuals with the disease are understandably anxious for as definitive information on prognosis as possible.

Until very recently there was little real possibility, although continuing hope, that survival times in the disease could be increased, with a cure an even more distant prospect. Whilst individuals with the disease have felt that, on occasion, their efforts at analysing and finding a therapeutic regimen for their own MND/ALS had prolonged their quantity and quality of life, most scientists have been sceptical about those claims because of individual variability in the course of the disease, and because of the usual absence of effective 'control subjects' against which the success of the therapeutic regime could be measured. However, following many desperate and hitherto abortive attempts, both through clinical trials and through individual clinical initiatives, to arrest or slow the disease with a wide range of agents, a number of clinical trials have now been yielding unexpectedly positive results. With the normally intractable and usually brutally consistent progression of the disease, any factor which appears to have even modest effects on its progress is both unexpected and encouraging.

The most plausible therapeutic possibilities, at least from the point of view of conventional science, have been those based on assumed causal mechanisms. For example, the genetic findings so far imply that neurological damage is partly sustained in the disease through a range of oxidation processes accelerated by defective genes. Therefore, it seems reasonable to pursue therapies which have anti-oxidant properties – possibly through vitamin and mineral regimes. However, there is little evidence that the damage already sustained would be redressed in any way by such regimes, not only because of the problems of targeting to damaged areas, but also because the damage is structural and continuing. None the less, for general health a strongly anti-oxidant-based diet is often recommended, and thus on those grounds alone might be continued. It appears, however, that much more work needs to be undertaken on how and in what ways specific genetic defects could be remedied to be confident of affecting the outcome of the disease.

More immediately promising therapies which might slow the course of MND/ALS are largely centred on two rather different approaches. The first of these is based on the role of neurotrophic factors in the disease. The relationship of these factors to each other is complex, and their absence appears to produce very specific pathologies in the nervous system in each case. None the less, the belief (and hope) has been that if one or more, or a specific combination, of such growth factors could be reintroduced into the nervous systems of people with MND/ALS, then further deterioration might be prevented to the remaining motor neurones, thus slowing down or even halting the disease at its present level, or, far more optimistically, leading to some regeneration of nervous tissue and thus the regaining of lost muscular control.

An increasing range of neurotrophic factors has been identified, and the main problems have been how to synthesise and reproduce these growth factors with sufficient purity and in sufficient quantity, what combination of them might be most appropriate, and how best to deliver them to the nervous system so that they might be most effective. Commercial pharmaceutical companies have played a leading part in the development of these neurotrophic factors to the point of clinical intervention, usually through recombinant genetic engineering techniques, and correspondingly over the last four years there has been a rapidly increasing number of clinical trials on such substances. The possible effectiveness of such factors as GDNF (glial-derived neurotrophic factor); CNTF (ciliary neurotrophic factor); BDNF (brain-derived neurotrophic factor), and even more recently others, has led to great pressure from people with MND/ALS and patient-based organisations, especially in the United States, not only for accelerated clinical trial procedures, but also for the early release of these agents for physicians and individuals to use on a compassionate basis.

The second major avenue along which there are promising therapeutic developments is that related to managing some of the problematic effects of what we described above as excitotoxity in the nervous system, and particularly managing excess glutamate and its consequences. An early controlled trial on one factor (riluzole – trade name Rilutek) with known properties affecting glutamate, produced – in MND/ALS terms – the striking finding that a statistically significant number of people with the disease receiving this factor had enhanced survival times of approximately three months more than those not receiving it. A range of findings have emerged from later trials, but the majority have indicated some positive results. This drug is now licensed for regular clinical use in a number of countries. Another factor (gabapentin – trade name Neurontin) has been shown to have a significant effect on glutamate in animal studies and preliminary clinical trials, and further trials of this factor are underway. Additional possibilities for the control of glutamate are under development.

The various individual strategies through which therapeutic options might be offered raise a multitude of putative combinations of drugs which could slow the course of MND/ALS. It is unlikely that all these can be formally evaluated quickly, given cost and resource issues, and thus there is considerable debate as to how best to proceed, especially in the light of the pressure from people with the disease for early release of drugs for individual use. We discuss these issues further in Chapter 5. There is currently a sense of optimism, even considerable excitement, about the possibilities which are now being developed and tested which may slow down – even marginally – the progression of MND/ALS. However, it is important to focus on the issues involved in the daily management of the many profoundly difficult symptoms of the disease which, for the foreseeable future, will be at the heart of most people's lives with the condition.

A range of other symptoms may require simultaneous management by a combination of drugs, physical therapies and lifestyle changes, including: continence problems – although these may be linked more to age related or other factors not directly attributable to MND/ALS; perhaps dysautonomia – cold, swollen feet and toes, and sometimes hands and fingers; fatigue – where recovery of previous strength or mobility is not obtained even by substantial rest; and sleep disorders.

Perhaps the most difficult set of issues to manage in every way are those concerned with bulbar symptoms – especially eating, drinking, swallowing (with potential problems over choking), excess salivation and mucus production, as well as voice production. In addition, what is usually described as emotional lability is often a problem – that is continuing (and what others would consider as inappropriate) weeping or laughing, or transitions between the two. Although not all of these symptoms necessarily occur together, to manage each one of them often requires a combination of personal determination and attention, technical expertise, experience, and often the assistance of others in both the formal and informal health care domains. A difficulty in swallowing combined with managing salivation is one of the most socially as well as medically difficult problems to contain. Such symptoms, allied with communicative difficulties as voice production becomes difficult and perhaps impossible by 'natural' means, present all concerned with MND/ALS with a particularly profound set of issues in which to engage in daily life.

As the disease progresses, it is likely that there will be an almost exponential increase in aids and equipment to assist in the management of the increasing and wide range of symptoms. This equipment may include: special beds, static chairs or wheelchairs; lifts and assistive devices for standing or bracing the body or neck; communication aids and equipment for assisting eating, drinking, swallowing or breathing; as well as many other possible pieces of equipment.

As the disease becomes very advanced there are a further set of critical issues to be faced in managing the disease, especially in relation to nutrition and respiration. In particular, there are issues of how, where and on what basis to ensure the comfort and well-being of the person with MND/ALS – and of those close to them – as well as how to manage the dying process. As we discuss in Chapter 6, there are now many complicated issues arising in relation to the possible maintenance of life of people with advanced MND/ALS. It is feasible, through the use of ventilators and a range of other devices, to assist breathing artificially for people with MND/ALS for some time – perhaps several years – after they would otherwise have died through respiratory failure. In addition, a variety of feeding techniques make it viable to maintain nutritional bodily integrity for lengthy periods after feeding by mouth has become too problematic. Such issues raise profound personal, social and ethical – as well as medical – concerns. Indeed, it should be noted that medical practices in relation to both assisted breathing and robust nutritional interventions are very different in different parts of the world. In Britain, and many countries in Europe, it is not usually a medically recommended, approved or supported option to have mechanical ventilation in the very advanced stages of the disease, and robust nutritional interventions are far less recommended unless they are for symptomatic or palliative purposes. The traditions in North America and Japan are very different and an increasing number of people with MND/ALS are using substantial ventilator support to maintain life.

Thus, the management of MND/ALS is a complex and multi-faceted process, which is both increasingly technical, on the one hand, but also, on the other hand, involves choices, issues and concerns which are of an intensely personal nature. Furthermore, the pace at which the symptoms of the disease can multiply and develop constantly places an onus on the person with MND/ALS, as well as those informally and formally assisting them, to adapt at speed to new and generally more problematic difficulties. Most formal health-care systems are not geared to managing the developing trajectory of such a disease with any great success, and thus there are frequently tensions which arise in meshing together the needs of the person with MND/ALS and formal health care support and resources. In this respect, extensive health care teams consisting of many professions are, in principle, necessary for the management of the problems of MND/ALS, and are now becoming *de rigueur* amongst health care providers. However, the almost incredible array of symptomatic problems which people with the disease can present highlights any deficiencies in the coordination as well as in the skills of professional health care staff.

In the light of major difficulties for patients over many years, increasingly patient-based voluntary organisations such as the Motor Neurone Disease Association (MNDA) in Britain, and the Amyotrophic Lateral Sclerosis Association (ALSA) in the United States, have either provided a virtually alternative formal health care service themselves for people with MND/ALS, or are providing funds and other support (as well as using considerable and vociferous pressure) to enhance the services of national and local health care providers. Other voluntary organisations, such as Monitor in Britain, have provided additional local services specifically for people with MND/ALS, as well as themselves acting to press for changes in the management of the disease.

None the less, whatever level of support is provided through statutory or voluntary health providers or other organisations, in

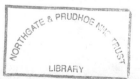

the end, as we note throughout this text, the main burden of the disease is likely to fall on the people with the disease and, most particularly, informal carers – family and friends.

BALANCING THE MEDICAL, SOCIAL AND PERSONAL IN MND/ALS

Without exaggeration it can be said that MND/ALS presents a major challenge to all those who are involved with people with the disease (Cobb and Hamera 1986). As a disease, it falls within the domain of science-based medicine to manage it formally in the Western world. However, it raises issues which go well beyond the current reach of science for doctors, nurses, physiotherapists and all the other professional staff who may be involved, and in which personal as well as professional beliefs, practices and experiences about the meaning – and management – of life and death are at the core. The remainder of this book is essentially about the relationship between the world of science-based medicine, and those who practice in or are close to it, and those people with the disease, their families and friends, as they try to make sense of what is happening to them as a profound personal and social experience.

Chapter 2

Motor neurone disease in the context of life
Experiencing onset and diagnosis

'NORMAL' AGEING AND MOTOR NEURONE DISEASE

The disentangling of the effects of ageing from those associated with the presence of a particular and very serious medical condition is not always an easy process for those intricately and personally bound up with both. Personal as well as social expectations of being older (let alone being old) often appear to focus on the increasing extent to which the physical body cannot function as it used to do, and on the increasing array of everyday symptoms which may be associated with the longer-term wear and tear of a lifetime's experiences and traumas. Such general understandings make it problematic initially for many people to work out what domain to place their symptoms in – that of the anticipated and 'normal' problems of an ageing body, or that of the untoward and abnormal onset of a potentially serious disease. The issue is how the identification occurs of what subsequently prove to be those special symptoms which, put together in a particular order within a particular life history by (usually) medical men, mean 'motor neurone disease'.

Of course both symptoms and disease are placed not so much in the context of the ageing body as a purely physical and abstract entity, but in the framework of *our own individual* bodies within our usual settings and with the people with whom we interact. We know our bodies both through our perception of them, and through other people's recognition and understanding of us through them. Bourdieu's (1984) idea of the 'habitus' is a useful way of conceptualising this issue, in thinking how older people might first discern the untoward beginnings of something like MND/ALS in their bodies, discriminating that from routine, expected and everyday ways in which their bodies have always operated. He argues that it (the habitus) is apparent:

> [in] the most automatic gestures [and] the apparently most insignificant techniques of the body – ways of walking or blowing one's nose – and engage[s] the most fundamental principles of construction and evaluation of the social world.
>
> (1984: 466)

The 'habitus' is essentially a socially based framework of practices which is deeply ingrained in people; indeed, 'the habitus is located within the body and affects every aspect of human embodiment' (Shilling 1993: 129). The importance of this idea is that it indicates a principle of which everyone knows the practice. That is, that your social position, experiences and background over a lifetime, conditions – Bourdieu might say determines – the nuances of the ways in which you manage your body, understand it, and how you present it to others. In this respect, it is perhaps not surprising that it may prove difficult for a person to determine the salience of what proves to be an initially modest physical symptom of MND/ALS which may already fit, in part, the complexities of their 'habitus'. In addition, the idea of 'habitus' may assist in understanding how the worlds of physician and the patient as person both differ, and can lead – at least at first – to problems in mutual understanding and communication over such symptoms. The physician's world is one in which, from a scientific point of view, the interpretation of bodily symptoms takes place in the context of a global and universal human biology and taxonomy of disease, whilst from the point of view of the patient symptoms are personal, local and social – and are indeed perceived in and through their own 'habitus'. The multiple implications of this view are now explored in relation to the onset and diagnosis of MND/ALS.

THE INITIAL PRESENTATION OF SYMPTOMS

The initial visibility of what in retrospect proves to be the forerunner symptoms of a serious condition are very variable as they fade into and out of the ordinary symptomatic vagaries of everyday life – indeed often just feature as part of the person's 'habitus'. They sometimes just slot into some of the particular characteristics through which people define themselves as, for example, clumsy or unfit. For instance, Colin notes how for a considerable period of time he did not recognise his problems as serious at all:

Looking back now the first signs were that my hands and arms seemed to be getting weaker, I dropped things, and it was difficult to do up buttons and so on. At the time this did not really worry me. I have always been a bit of a clumsy person, and my family often remarked on this – you know bumping into things, and dropping things. It seemed a bit worse but I thought, 'What can you expect at my time of life?' In any case we all have to make adjustments as we grow older. We are not what we were!

His condition only came to the attention of the formal health-care system when a friend came round to see him, and suggested that he really ought to see a doctor because, to the friend, his weakness appeared as more than just one of those signs of growing older. Then, after a referral from his GP, Colin went through a whole series of orthopaedic investigations and operations for a compressed nerve, and even a tendon transplant to relieve what was by now considered to be a 'dropped wrist'.

Jeff was another person who did not initially perceive his symptoms as anything special or significant:

I had been a cyclist all my life and sometimes rode for two hundred miles or so a day for several days at a time, and regularly used to ride between fifty and a hundred miles. But due to pressure at work I had virtually had to give up cycling, and over several months had not done much at all. It was just when I started again that I had some weakness in my legs, and I thought that it was understandable because I hadn't ridden for so long. My immediate thought was to get fit, and do extra training, not only on the bike, but at home on weights. This seemed to work initially, and probably I did get fitter, although I still felt that there was some kind of problem. But I just put that down to being too ambitious, and that I should really scale down my riding. Actually in conversation with my GP early on about something else I just mentioned the problem, but he seemed to think of the same solution to it that I did – I needed to get fit again.

It was only later when Jeff was on a short cycling tour, and found to his embarrassment and shock that he could not lift his leg over a style and had to get someone to do this for him, that he began to become concerned. The final symptom which sped him though the medical system and led to his diagnosis of MND/ALS was a pronounced deterioration in his speech, which he felt meant he could not carry out his job in local government.

Jack found a visit to his local pub led to unanticipated symptoms, and eventually to an innovative way to deal with one of the particularly socially stigmatised symptoms of the disease:

> After leaving the pub my voice became slurred; this happened quite suddenly. My first thought was a build up of alcohol, my second thought was that I had loose dentures. So I started drinking slimline tonic, and I ordered and got new dentures. However 'a new slimline Jack' still slurred his speech. I visited the doctor; he said that perhaps I had had a slight stroke. I left it at that for the time being. Going out at this time I wore a self-made badge saying 'I'm not drunk, it's your evil mind'. This way I got a laugh instead of curiosity. However, I knew there was something that needed a further look, and when I went for a thorough examination at the hospital they told me I had motor neurone disease.

Jack epitomises, in his matter-of-fact way, the wide range of ways in which symptoms might be explained as part of a current lifestyle, and also how even at a relatively early stage socially problematic situations may arise.

For Tom, an older man, it was the persistent concerns of others which eventually led to his symptoms being appropriately diagnosed. His daughter recounts:

> My father had difficulty raising his right arm. After discussions with him I took him to the doctor who diagnosed a frozen shoulder and told him it would clear up in eighteen months. I personally spoke to the doctor about him because I felt that something else was wrong, but I was assured that there was nothing to worry about. At this time even his friends would ask 'What is wrong with Tom?' Then an X-ray of his shoulder revealed he had slight arthritis, but then my father's condition worsened to the point where he couldn't get out of the bath unaided or put on his jacket himself. His left arm was affected, and he was having difficulty shaving. I took him to a physiotherapist who thought he might have a trapped nerve, but not a frozen shoulder – she also thought he might have had a minor

stroke. I then insisted that the GP refer him to someone else, and that's when he went to see the neurologist, and we learnt he probably had MND.

Given the prevalence of rheumatoid arthritis at older ages (nearly 50 per cent of people over sixty-five will have some symptoms of this disease (Jette 1996: 95)) this explanation of muscular or movement difficulties in older people is not an unexpected one, and statistically is almost certainly a correct diagnosis for the majority of such cases. However Tom's situation does highlight the difficulties of the parties to this diagnostic transaction, for the GP was technically correct in diagnosing arthritis, whilst Tom's daughter 'knew' that something more was wrong. Such a situation occurs in relation to other chronic diseases where once diagnosed such a disease is often used medically to explain *all* other symptoms (Robinson 1988), especially where chronic diseases – perhaps almost by definition – are seen as having systemic effects.

For other people the transition from first symptoms through to diagnosis may be relatively quick. This is not only because, particularly in older persons, the pre-existing build up of neuronal damage may produce a rapidly accelerated pattern of symptoms following the first symptom, but the nature of the symptoms themselves may produce relatively dramatic imperatives for social and medical action. Pam's description of her husband's symptoms shows how such a pathway into diagnosis operates:

My husband has always been a pretty fit man, indeed he prided himself on how he looked after his body. Then I noticed that he started stumbling frequently; he joked about it at first, but both he and I realised after a few days that this was something serious for he was having big difficulties at home just walking around without losing his balance. Our GP immediately sent us to the neurologist after a quick examination, and even before we had seen the neurologist, my husband's condition had got far worse. The neurologist said he thought he might know what was wrong but wanted to do some further tests. Looking back it was the speed of the changes in my husband that was so striking; we just had to do something about it.

These particular accounts, as almost all the others on which this analysis is based, emphasise not only the degree to which symptoms are always contextualised by reference to the everyday settings in which they occur, but also indicate their irredeemably social nature. That is that symptoms, as signs of health problems, and in these cases as the first signs of MND/ALS, are perceived, negotiated and acted upon in the light of observations and comments by others and through interactions with them. They demonstrate that body movements, body rhythms and body processes are not only the ways in which we recognise ourselves, but also how we are recognised by others. Changes in them are the way that both parties (self and others) realise that something is wrong or problematic and that they may be signs of abnormality, disease or ill-health requiring medical intervention.

Adamson argues that individuals, through reflecting on such changes, are brought into a state of what she calls existential uncertainty that:

> is that form of uncertainty which is experienced privately by the individual patient upon the realisation that the future life of his or her mind, body and self is in jeopardy.
>
> (1997: 134)

The logical way to proceed in this situation, given the central position of scientific medicine in the management of actual or potential illness, is to attempt a resolution to this kind of uncertainty through medical advice. Thus, seeking medical confirmation of these provisional judgements already made is the next stage in this process. The 'communication of the diagnosis' is the formal point at which the fears, hopes and curiosities aroused by those provisional judgements are made manifest in a medical setting. However, in Adamson's terms, as we shall argue, existential uncertainty for the individual with MND/ALS is not necessarily relieved at all by engagement with clinical medicine, and the communication of the diagnosis, far from reducing that uncertainty, may increase it.

COMMUNICATING THE DIAGNOSIS OF MND/ALS

Not only has 'communication' become one of the key words in the medical lexicon in very recent years, but rhetoric about the problems caused by bad communication on the one hand, or the possibilities created by good communication on the other has become a standard feature of discussions about the doctor–patient relationship. Nowhere have these issues been debated more widely than in relation to the communication of diagnoses by doctors to patients. This is an understandable development for a number of reasons. First, diagnosis in a real sense is prognosis, for the identification and naming of a condition implies the future course of that condition, as well as possible therapeutic interventions in that course. Thus, the communication of the diagnosis is the crucial point at which such information can be relayed to the patient. Second, for both parties (patient and doctor) there is likely to have been a lengthy period of inquiry, investigation, uncertainty and anxiety preceding the public naming of the disease to the patient. The revelation of the disease is therefore a culmination of this process leading to the replacement (in principle) of uncertainly by certainty, and the bringing in of the patient to the community of those whose problems are now legitimately medical. Third, at this point and thereafter, the doctor–patient relationship changes for (again in principle) it ceases to be one of clinical and intellectual investigative work to detect which unknown disease the patient has and becomes one of managing a known disease – or, in more appropriate terms, managing a patient with a known disease.

In the case of MND/ALS there are two added complications – for both doctors and patients – in addition to what might be seen as the usual complexities which attend the communication of medical diagnoses. First, in the vast majority of cases, MND/ALS is fatal within a relatively short period of time – three to five years. Second, there is still only a very modest repertoire of interventions which *might* slow down the course of the disease marginally, but still with a fatal outcome as a result. Thus, a major difficulty for both parties is that the communication of the diagnosis increases certainty, but it also increases the certainty of death with no curative mitigation. For the patients and their relatives seeking curative hope, therefore, at present none can be given biomedically. For the doctors, whose practices have been built on the promise of curative medicine, other grounds have to be sought on which to manage their relationship with these patients.

A further particular difficulty in relation to following up effectively the communication of the diagnosis lies in the history of the neurological enterprise, which has always focused more on unravelling the diagnostic puzzle that attends the mysteries of the brain and nervous system than on the day-to-day management of patients with the resulting diagnoses. Although this pattern is now changing with the rapid spread of neurologically based rehabilitation programmes in which those with a dying trajectory may also often participate, the intractability of most neurological conditions, including MND/ALS, to the conventional armoury of curative medicine still casts a considerable shadow over how to discuss the future with patients.

Despite the advent of guidelines, training courses, extensive commentaries and advice from august sources on the management of the communication of diagnoses, the ways in which such communication is undertaken in relation to MND/ALS, in relation to other conditions, appears to be remarkable for its local variations, and in general for its resistance to attempts to introduce more uniform practices. This situation arises partly through the protection of local clinical autonomy and partly through the differential experience and backgrounds of neurologists in particular; also, in part, through the balance which is struck locally between the diagnosis and management of patients, and, finally, through the personal preferences and concerns of neurologists and their capacities to manage relationships with dying people.

A triumphalist approach to the communication of the diagnosis of MND/ALS still appears in some quarters as a lengthy and no doubt contentious discussion about diagnostic possibilities between doctors that in the end results in a definitive diagnosis which all (the doctors) accept. Jane reports that her mother had spent several weeks in a leading neurological centre and:

> although she was very shocked and confused by the whole thing, and was not aware of the fate that awaited her, she kept saying that a large number of doctors had examined her from Germany and America and other places, and none of them seemed to know what was wrong with her . . . She then told me how, finally, a Dr X had 'triumphed over the other doctors' and had finally discovered what she had. He was apparently held in awe by the other doctors, and 'he seemed very pleased with himself'. She was not told the specific diagnosis herself, but a staff nurse came in later to tell her that something had happened to her that had caused weakness on one side of her body, and that 'in a year or so she would have another shock' and the other side of her body would be affected.

Given the myriad of often obscure and rare neurological conditions, and the need for sophisticated intellectual application to the interpretation of conflicting signs and symptoms, it is possible to understand the doctors' pleasure at such an outcome. At the same time, it is also possible that the patient appreciates this level of application and the definitive (as opposed to an imprecise) outcome. None the less, there is a common view amongst neurologists, expressed by Bradley, that the diagnosis of MND/ALS:

> In clinical terms . . . [is] easy in most cases, even for the neurologist with relatively limited experience.
>
> (1994: 27)

The problem is precisely that, as yet, such a diagnosis is a clinical one, with relatively little definitive laboratory or other objective physiological data to support it categorically. Thus, even if the neurologist is personally certain of the diagnosis there is often a lengthy process of formal investigation to eliminate other marginally possible diagnoses, not least because the known prognosis of MND/ALS is so poor. Bradley notes that whereas in the United States an exhaustive series of tests is often undertaken, which he believes are largely inappropriate given key clinical signs, in other countries no other investigation is undertaken other than what he calls the 'investigation of time' which should reveal the inexorable progression of the disease. The problem in relation to batteries of tests is that:

> They [physicians] sometimes get wrapped up in 'abnormal' test results and keep the patient unaware of the diagnosis even after many tests and return visits. The patient often becomes aware that the condition is serious, that it is progressively deteriorating, and that the doctor is concerned since all of these tests are being done. If the patient is not told anything, he or she may lose confidence in the doctor at this stage, and seek another or several other opinions. On the other side, it is not infrequent for the doctor to lack the confidence or perhaps the moral courage to tell the patient the diagnosis. Such a doctor will refer the patient [to another physician] without sharing the diagnosis.
>
> (1994: 23)

In Britain, from the accounts of people with MND/ALS drawn on for this analysis, lengthy catalogues of 'tests' are reported. Although, in part, these have occurred through initial incorrect referral to orthopaedic specialists, or to rheumatologists in particular, there is every reason to believe that the difficult dynamics of the diagnostic process described by Bradley are as applicable as in the United States. None the less, whatever the process by which the diagnosis is reached the doctors have only solved one of a patient's puzzles, and they may not be able to respond in such categorical ways to almost all the other puzzles which will now present themselves to a patient and their relatives. The puzzle of which disease it is has been solved, but the greater question of the quality of life of, and for, the patient and their relatives remains.

However, the case of Jane's mother raises other issues: most notably, and bluntly, how are people told that they are very likely to die in the near future? For some, the process did indeed occur bluntly, as this recollection by Dick of the communication of the diagnosis to his wife Elizabeth indicates:

Patient: What do you think it is Doctor?

Dr X: It seems to be one of three things. You have something amiss with your knee joint, you have something amiss with your back, you have Motor Neurone Disease.

Patient: Which one of the three do you suspect Doctor?

Dr X: I suspect Motor Neurone Disease.

Patient: What exactly is that Doctor?

Dr X: It is a disease that affects the muscles of the body.

Patient: Can you do anything about it?

Dr X: No, there is unfortunately no known cure.

Patient: Will it stop?

Dr X: No. It is progressive. However, go away and enjoy your holidays. I will have you into the hospital when you come back for further tests.

Patient: You have been pretty abrupt Doctor.

Dr X: You asked me for the truth and I have told you.

This was my wife's and my first indication of the disease. It had a very traumatic effect on my wife because of the lack of any reassurance. This made her holiday very sad.

Although many people wish accurate and clear information, and indeed wish to know 'the truth', the incisive and robust way in which this doctor communicated the diagnosis self-evidently short-circuits what many might regard as a necessary sensitivity to the patient's world. Rachel had a similar kind of experience, but in a different setting

[After three days of tests in hospital] the next day my husband joined me and waited for Dr X [the consultant neurologist] to give us his diagnosis. When we were admitted to his domain we sat in the centre of the room with Dr X, virtually surrounded by Dr Y, a Sister, the Occupational Therapist, the Speech Therapist, the Physiotherapist and four students – and in front of them all he gave me a death sentence. He said that he would give me the good news first which was that I had no brain tumour, but that what I had got was a form of palsy – there was no known cause and no known cure. When my husband said that we were planning to go to Australia in two years time, Dr X said 'You can forget that. Go now, you won't be going then'.

We left the . . . hospital in the depths of despair not knowing what to do or where to turn. We had no suspicion that my illness was terminal as, apart from the speech and swallowing difficulties, I was apparently in perfect health. We were offered nothing as there is no known cure and felt that a death sentence could have been delivered with some compassion, and certainly not in front of so many strangers.

The immediacy with which Elizabeth and Rachel and their partners understood the implications of their diagnosis is not always the pattern as descriptions of MND/ALS by the doctor may be wrapped in a more complex language. For example, in the case of Bill receiving his diagnosis with his daughter she reports that:

Although [following several days of tests] Dr X had been very open and straightforward in his explanation of the disease, Dad virtually took in nothing of what he said. He was in a state of nervous tension, overawed by the occasion and the fear that he would be kept in for further tests. He sat rigid. I held his hand throughout after the word 'irreversible' . . . and I knew he wasn't taking in much. Part of this was due to the 'medical' language being used (he had had little schooling) e.g. 'irreversible', 'neurone', 'prognosis', 'degenerative', 'premature wearing out', 'transmission' and so on.

In this case, as in many others, the immediate relative was taken aside and given a more detailed and practical account of what the implications were of the diagnosis. Bill's daughter was told that she urgently had to make plans for future nursing care as soon her father would not be able to walk at all, and that he almost certainly had little more than two years to live.

The role of relatives in the communication of the diagnosis is a complex and often very burdensome one. With a diagnosis such as

MND/ALS it appears very infrequently that the person is told alone
– except 'by accident', or through sets of relatively unusual circumstances. The more usual pattern is either for the person to be told
with a partner or son or daughter, or for that relative to be told
alone first. Margaret, in effect, pre-empted what the consultant
might have done, but this left her with a continuing problem as to
when and how to tell her husband:

> Whilst Eric was in the examination room I asked the consultant
> 'Does it kill?' To this day I don't know what prompted me to ask,
> and then I got the prognosis and not the diagnosis . . . the most
> difficult thing I have ever done was to try and appear normal to
> Eric within minutes of receiving the prognosis, and to invent a
> conversation between the consultant and myself which would
> satisfy Eric. The following day, whilst Eric was out, I phoned
> close family on both sides and close friends and told them . . . I
> have always believed, and still do, that the terminally ill should
> be told so that they may sort out their affairs so that all is
> smooth sailing for those left behind, [rather than] by the time
> they know, without being told, they are too ill to do anything
> about it. I didn't tell Eric, I suppose because the consultant
> hadn't and I felt duty bound to follow his lead. I did intend to
> tell him when he was worse but not too ill. [For almost a year]
> until he found out, it was terribly difficult to appear cheerful and
> reassuring but somehow one finds the strength to do what has to
> be done.

Particularly for older couples, who have faced many of life's difficulties together, there is resistance to the idea that one of them –
usually the partner without MND/ALS – should receive the news
first. Indeed, for couples who have prided themselves on not
keeping secrets from each other, the often strongly held view of a
consultant that one of them and not the other should receive the
news first presents a major additional problem and raises profound
personal and ethical issues for the couple. It is not clear why consul-
tants may take this particular view, although it is common in
relation to other serious conditions (Robinson 1988). However, it
seems to be based on a perspective that serious diseases are
emotionally disabling for the patient, but far less so for their relatives, and that it is an easier task (for the doctor?) that the news be
broken by a relative to the patient. In Jackie's case she was left in
disarray by the doctor's news to her alone, but then he redeemed

himself (for her) for he rescued the situation a few days later by informing her husband:

> [After tests in the hospital] the following day on my way to visit him I saw a consultant (after asking previously to talk to someone about how long before he completely loses the use of his legs) who told me that he had only 6 months to 2 years to live, and it was MND. I had never heard of this or had any idea about it. I then had to visit Joe and be cheerful for an hour when my heart was breaking up (we had had 32 years of happy married life and loved each other dearly). Can you imagine how I felt. Thank goodness my son was with me as otherwise I did not know how I should have driven the 20 miles home. I fetched him home at the end of August and we were asked to go back for a consultation in the second week of September. I could not tell him [her husband] what had been said to me previously. The consultant then told Joe what he had and that they do not know what causes it and there was nothing at all they could do for him.

Some partners resist robustly the view that they should be separated when the diagnosis is communicated, although this does not necessarily make the situation much more bearable as in this case:

> I had no idea of what might be wrong with my husband, as I had never heard of MND . . . the Doctor said tests would be made, and if it was the spine then he may be able to help but if not, then there would be nothing he could do. At that moment I made it very clear that whatever the diagnosis my husband or I had to be together, we fought all our battles together. After my husband had had the tests, I received a telephone call from the ward sister early afternoon to see the Doctor half an hour before visiting time. I died a thousand times during those 4 hours. When I got to the hospital and whilst I was waiting, I heard the Doctor ask if I was on my own, he then asked to talk to me without my husband. I had to insist my husband and I must be together. We were told why Fred was experiencing the problems which were [particularly] troublesome for his job, but not their very seriousness. I had to ask if this condition had a name, but then we didn't realise the horror of what the future was going to be. Until I secretly read about it in the library. I was so devastated I went to bed that night and couldn't sleep. Even to this day, four years later, I still have sleep problems.

Although, medically, the communication of such a diagnosis is often considered to be between the doctor, frequently with other members of their team, and the person with MND/ALS and/or their partner, son or daughter, in many cases there are other complications to this process. In particular, for the person and partner there are a set of what might be called 'domino communications' to consider as difficult decisions are made about how far and when the diagnostic knowledge should cascade down to other relatives or friends. In the case of Michael it was exceptionally difficult as he sought to control the process:

> It was many months before I informed members of my and Vivian's [his wife, who had been diagnosed with MND] families of the prognosis. This was deliberate as I wished to tell them directly rather than by letter from the Middle East. Thus it was not until my next annual leave that I was able to tell Vivian's sisters and my own brothers and sisters. I also considered that Richard [his son] had the right to know, he then being twenty-two years of age, in case anything should happen to me, but I thought that Sophie [his daughter], at seventeen, did not need to know for the time being. However, the manner in which Richard was to learn of his mother's illness was extremely unfortunate, and most distressing for him, for it did not occur in the way I had planned, for it was just blurted out over the telephone by one of my relatives... Naturally this was a very severe shock to Richard ... and I was very distressed when I learned that he had been told in this way, and to this day I have a sense of guilt on that account.

The management of this kind of communicative process is extremely problematic within families, not only in determining how and when the telling occurs, but in attempting to gauge the response of family members. In Michael and Richard's case all three elements went astray through a series of miscalculations. In such situations, part of the miscalculation is the view that the dissemination of information can be controlled in a carefully calculated way, as it were by (often unspoken) personal authority. However, as in Richard's case, sources of information may be multiple and resistant to easy management. In medical situations, although a person's medical notes may frequently record diagnostically incriminating information about MND/ALS, it is often assumed that only the consultant can inform the person of the diagnosis, or may already have done so. Communicative 'mishaps' occur in this situation through an unwitting reading aloud of the notes by nursing or other staff or even, as in this case, by Colin surreptitiously having a sight of his notes:

Up to this point [in a lengthy medical investigation of his problems] there had been no mention of MND/ALS. In fact I had never heard of it . . . [however] during a physiotherapy session, the physiotherapist had to leave the room for another call. Being of an inquisitive nature I ventured to look at my medical notes left on the table. There for the first time I saw the name MND . . . I did not say anything at the time but on my way home I called into my local library and looked up MND in the medical books. There I learnt for the first time the full implications of MND, notably the point that most patients gradually get weaker all over their body and then usually die within 3 to 4 years. Needless to say I went home in a daze that evening. I felt I could not tell my wife as it all seemed so unreal. Here I was a very fit person, playing regular sport, soccer, squash, golf every week. How could I possibly die within 3 years?

At least for some, there was relief at the point of communication of the diagnosis for, after a period of uncertainty, the naming of the disease and the placing of it firmly within the repertory of medicine was reassuring. However, such reassurance did not usually last long:

When it was diagnosed that I had MND, the consultant didn't give me any details about the illness and of that I am glad. He did, however, tell my wife of some of the effects of the condition adding that there would be no point in us seeing him again. [In retrospect] the diagnosis was somewhat of a relief because I had known that I was 'really' poorly but just with what I had no idea, I don't quite think that I had heard of MND. I knew it was serious and it upset me, but then that was before I gradually learned of the unpleasant details.

For others, too, some feeling of relief was not an uncommon experience as they were taken through the diagnostic process and were anxious for a clear medical assessment. However, other major issues may surface in this situation and overwhelm any sense of relief. As Joan points out:

[When my husband was diagnosed as having MND/ALS] the

diagnosis was communicated by the neurologist. It was given to me in his office, and to my husband whilst he was still laying undressed on his couch! [However] my husband was not told the exact details of his illness, and I was told to break things to him gently. No one suspected the diagnosis before we saw the neurologist, and apart from knowing that David Niven had died from an unknown disease, we had never heard of MND/ALS. The diagnosis was a shock, but my husband, not knowing the details saw it as a relief. Our immediate response was one of disbelief. My husband was a very fit person, who watched his health, this sort of illness only happened to other people. I think we both felt very bitter. No support at all was offered at the time of diagnosis from anybody, we had to seek out the support and help we eventually got. The neurologist in reply to my question, 'Will we be seeing you again?' said, 'What is the point, how will he get here?' He spoke to me just like telling someone they had to have a tooth out, he just seemed indifferent to our problem. Until I asked him, after I had gathered my 'wits' together, he did not even tell me what the illness was called.

This is not a universal view, however, for knowing the terminal nature of the diagnosis at once pre-empts what one person feels would be a stage-by-stage accommodation to the disease and its end result. Julie said:

My husband died seven years after it [MND] was diagnosed . . . I felt towards the end, and thinking back on when the consultant told me, 'Why did they have to tell me then? We could have coped better if we could have taken it a stage at a time.'

Perhaps this just emphasises the wide range of ways of managing news about a terminal diagnosis, and the difficulty of predicting what that approach might be in other people. In this respect, few people have had the experience of being given such a diagnosis themselves more than once, and even if they have been informed before about such a diagnosis in someone close to them, the circumstances, and probably the consequences, are likely to have been very different.

In a condition with a similar prognosis to MND/ALS, Salander *et al.* (1996) found that the current vogue for clear and detailed information about the prognosis and consequences of the disease at the outset was not welcomed by many patients they studied. Moreover, in relation to this condition – a malignant brain tumour – doctors generally appeared to discuss the prognosis in an ambiguous and vague way. Salander *et al.* argue that:

> The vagueness [of the doctor about the implications of the diagnosis] may be a conscious or subconscious adjustment to the patient's need for a transitional area. It might be that when the doctor informs the patient about the diagnosis with warmth and clarity, s/he is giving a substantial contribution to the building of a transitional area between him/herself and the patient as an area where the patient can create protection and hope.
>
> (1996: 994)

In this respect the key to assisting patients to manage this particular diagnosis:

> [was not] just a matter of saying 'cancer' or 'tumour', but rather of implementing a situation that makes it possible for the patient to create his/her essential illusion . . . It is very much a question of being sensitive to the patient's reconstructed reality . . . [thus] the patient is aware of the situation but the avoidance isolates this knowledge which facilitates a view of the situation built on the creative protecting process.

The construction of hope in the face of terminal diagnosis, 'the essential illusion' to which Salander *et al.* refer, is not in their terms a problematic solution to the management of the diagnosis by patients, and thus should not be considered as such by doctors. Indeed, it is quite the contrary. Rather than being seen as a pathological denial of the disease or its terminal nature, it is a way of managing the existential uncertainty (Adamson 1997) to which we referred earlier, and placing this in the more familiar and comforting surroundings of a patient's 'habitus', and his or her existing life world. Such a process is hard work and requires information, thoughts, actions and feelings which may owe relatively little to scientific medicine, and perhaps even less to the detail of the formal information about the disease and its prognosis which might be given at the outset. For those with MND/ALS this process is especially difficult and is explored in Chapters 3 and 4.

A greater difficulty does exist however for relatives of people given a diagnosis of a terminal illness, as accounts above make clear. Salander *et al.* point to this phenomenon in their study, which included the partners of those with a malignant brain tumour:

> They were affected by the psychological impact of the disease of their partners, but as they were not ill themselves, they did not have access to protection and hope [which might be constructed] from their own bodies. In this sense they stood aside, and reality remained overridden by insecurity and anxiety ... They [the patient and the partner] could not share a common view of the situation. One [the patient] ... brought reality together with hope and created illusion, the other [the partner] saw reality as mute reality. This is important ... to understand the exposed position of the partners. It was not uncommon that they felt divided between double loyalties: the loyalty to themselves and their own anxiety on the one hand, and to the patient and his/her illusion on the other.

Whilst the possibility of illusion, in the form of hope may, for various reasons, be more problematic to achieve in the case of MND/ALS, than in the case of those with malignant brain tumours, the position of relatives, especially partners, appears to be similar. Salander *et al.* implicitly argue that there are unfortunate paradoxes operating at the point of communication of the diagnosis as far as relatives are concerned, which appear to be present in the case of MND/ALS, as well as in the case of MS (Robinson 1988). For doctors, relatives and especially partners are often considered as rational, healthy, stable and supportive allies to whom, in preference to the patient, diagnoses should be communicated. In fact – and paradoxically – there is growing evidence that this is a mistaken view and often relatives, as the accounts in this chapter suggest, feel not only burdened with the diagnostic news, but are left with further difficult decisions about relaying this information to the person with MND/ALS.

MOVING BEYOND THE COMMUNICATION OF THE DIAGNOSIS

We have charted just some of the dimensions of the experience of MND/ALS from the point at which symptoms are just barely perceptible to the point at which the diagnosis of MND/ALS is communicated.

However, this way of phrasing the issue of when you now 'know' you have MND/ALS is in many respects very problematic. Diagnoses are not 'known' by people with serious diseases in the sense that is often inferred by doctors, or indeed especially inferred by medical texts – that is, as a body of medical (scientific) facts about diagnosis and prognosis – however sensitively they may be transmitted. It would be more appropriate to argue that diagnoses are 'experienced', rather than 'known', unless the former is considered as a definition of the latter. In this sense, for an individual, and for their family, a diagnosis is, in Bury's felicitous phrase (used in a different context), the result of 'continuously emerging meaning' (1988). Daily life with the disease itself constantly reworks what the diagnosis means – as symptoms change, as their consequences change, and as reflection on both occurs and recurs. In this respect, to put the point bluntly and controversially, the diagnosis is never 'communicated' in the form of an event; it is always in the process of being communicated. Thus, in the case of MND/ALS, the meaning of the diagnosis is constructed and reconstructed many times as the implications of this disease change from day to day and week to week. In the next chapters we explore these issues further.

Chapter 3

Reframing life and death with motor neurone disease
The quest to understand and manage the disease

RECONCILING MEDICAL AND PERSONAL AGENDAS

Adapting to, managing or coping with a difficult situation, such as that produced by the intrusion of a disease such as MND/ALS in someone's life, apparently requires accurate and detailed information about the diagnosis and its associated prognosis, as well as about any specific curative – or in the case of MND/ALS – palliative treatments. Indeed, at one level it does. However, such information is not a neutral commodity, particularly from the perspective of the person with the disease and their relatives. For whilst, in principle, such people do require accurate and detailed information, it is information as it relates not just to the disease with which they have been diagnosed, but specifically to their particular situation with all its nuances, special sets of circumstances and so on – in other words to *their* disease. This issue of *the* disease as against *their* disease is one which is troublesome for almost all relationships between those working within the framework of contemporary scientific medicine, and others who are subject to their ministrations.

Christiakis puts this issue in neat historical perspective in his analysis of the changing ways in which doctors and medical scientists have, since the nineteenth century, considered the relationship between the disease and the person. His views raise other important and salient questions about how people with MND/ALS and their relatives both do, and might, interact with the medical profession in their quest to understand and manage the condition. He notes how initially in the late nineteenth century:

> if two individuals were exposed to the same contagious element the one who had the 'firmer' constitution would have a more

favourable outcome. The prognoses of the two individuals would differ on the basis of individual factors distinct from the diagnosis itself. The two individuals would have in some sense different diseases.

(1997: 314)

Later patients were deemed to have the *same* disease in the sense there was:

> a cognitive shift toward the notion that disease had a discrete existence that was not only ontological and etiologic but also prognostic – that a disease had a 'natural course' that was 'typical'.

With this shift from the view that the particular characteristics or constitution of the individual person *were* the disease, and thus had to be addressed, to a view that the disease existed independently (as it were) of the person:

> there has been an ellipsis of prognosis. Prognosis is viewed as a simple extension of diagnosis, an extension typically not necessitating explicit consideration.

This position has then led to a problem for the diagnosis and prognosis of all conditions because with the emphasis on 'typicality', there always appear to be 'atypical' cases, which both confound the prognosis of 'typical' cases, and lead to a further search for variations of diseases, or even new diseases, for which a revised 'typicality' is assumed to exist.

In the case of MND/ALS, the 'typical' prognosis is clear – that is that following diagnosis around 60 per cent of people die within three years, and over 90 per cent within five years. In between diagnosis and death there will be a progressive loss of muscular control, which may be variable at first but which becomes increasingly similar as the course of the disease proceeds. However, whilst, by and large, doctors are working on the basis of such standardised clinically and epidemiologically driven data, patients (people with MND/ALS) are always working on the basis of their individual 'atypical' and personal agendas. These latter agendas are focused on the attempt to resolve existential uncertainty, as we noted in Chapter 2, and:

> Whereas existential uncertainty is resolved by an individual's

freely chosen actions, clinical uncertainty is a problem that invites a collective, intersubjectively verifiable solution.

(Adamson 1997: 153)

In this context, a major difficulty for people with MND/ALS in conversations with their doctors is that the latter are working within the bounds of standardised knowledge which is detached from such individual agendas, and thus have considerable professional – as well as scientific – difficulty in reaching out to address what they may see as highly personal, idiosyncratic or irrelevant concerns, especially when the 'typical' prognosis is so (scientifically) self-evident.

THE CHRONOLOGY OF TIME AND LIFE WITH MND/ALS

One of the most contentious and problematic areas, which exercises both patients and doctors about MND/ALS immediately following the communication of the diagnosis, is that of the quantity and quality of time left to the person with MND/ALS – and of course, by implication, to their relatives. The paradox is that although these questions are very frequently asked, and they are statistically and scientifically answerable with some precision by reference to scientific research on many 'typical' cases, at the same time, in personal terms they are almost completely unanswerable.

A simple chronology of time – for example, whether someone is told that they have two months or two years to live – is only marginally helpful information. Time has many dimensions of which linear time is only one, and indeed the only way that such stark information can be made to make personal sense is to rework that information into personal and social time. Is there time to search out all the possibilities that might slow down the disease? Is there time to achieve a myriad of personal and family objectives with family and friends? Is there time to see particular festivals – for example, Easter or Christmas? Is there time to celebrate at impending births and marriages, to be present at other key social events, or to commiserate at others' deaths? Is there time to reflect on the past, to come to terms with one's own situation, to reconcile oneself to others, and to construct as good a way as possible to leave life? On, a more mundane but equally important level, is there time to work out how to manage the progressive day-to-day difficulties of living with the disease?

In addition, there is the major issue of the quality of the quantity of time. Many life objectives involve doing something, making something or being active in some capacity. They involve a special commitment and a particular embodied presence which the course of MND/ALS may make difficult, or impossible, some time before death. No doctor is likely to know the particular construction that someone with MND/ALS, or their relatives, place on all these separate but interlocking dimensions of time. None the less, it is clear that they are expected to acknowledge their existence. For example Sheila said:

> While my husband was being taken to the examination room I just said to the consultant – I don't know why – 'Will it kill him?' He didn't answer. Then my husband was examined, came back and then sent away while the neurologist asked me to remain behind. He made me ask my question again and said 'Yes' and I then asked 'How long?' He said '2 years'. We could have been talking about the weather and how long rain had been forecast. I thanked him and left and invented a pack of lies to explain to my husband why I had been asked to stay behind. I know that doctors are dishing out death sentences all the time but they should remember how people receive them, and whilst I don't expect a lengthy discussion I would have hoped for some expression of sympathy, and a helpful reflection on the situation.

In this case, the 'medical fact' of likely death within a particular period was relayed honestly, accurately and clearly – even if very bluntly – but this was only part of the response that Sheila expected from her doctor. She expected the doctor to go beyond the facts, to empathise with her situation, in effect to be with her as another person – a supportive and expert friend – sharing her immediate concerns and dilemmas about what having two years to live meant to her and her husband.

There are additional issues in working out how best to manage what is often described by people with MND/ALS and their relatives as a 'death sentence', based on the chronology given by a doctor. Although the doctor is usually 'just' reporting the available best evidence from scientific data, at the same time he or she is not detached from that data, for it has been given their personal imprimatur, and the patient considers them not only as personally owning the data but also as, in a direct sense, being individually responsible for its production. In some situations, chronological life that is 'taken away' by doctors can also be 'given back' by them. For example Julie reports that:

> My husband returned to the hospital to see a specialist he saw originally, who had diagnosed arthritis. He [now] said my husband had MND/ALS. As my husband left the room to get dressed he told me my husband was a very sick man and had about 2 months to live. I did not tell my husband this, as he was now given an appointment to see a leading consultant neurologist, and he was delighted to think he was getting somewhere at last, and that the quality of his life would now be improved. This consultant told us (as we knew already) that there was no known treatment or cure for MND/ALS, but he would prescribe some muscle relaxing drugs to make my husband feel better, and that he could be helped to feel more comfortable. This time my husband asked the consultant the prognosis, and was told he would live 2–4 years. As this consultant was a neurologist, I felt very relieved that my husband was not now to die in 2 months time – presuming he knew more than the arthritis specialist.

Julie is hopefully, from her point of view, correctly relying on the judgement of what she regards as the more expert of the experts she has encountered, and perhaps even more important has received some positive support and assistance in relation to her husband's condition. In this respect it is the individual doctor, as a person, who is relaying this information, and thus has a duty – in the patient's eyes – to be with them through the coming months and years in meeting all the challenges of the prognosis. Jack has had a rather different experience, and puts his views with some feeling, in making a number of other telling comments:

> Summing up the whole experience, I must admit my main feeling was one of intense anger against the medical profession. For anyone over 70 to be told they have an incurable disease seems to me no worse than knowing we have had at least a biblical lifespan, and we're lucky to have had that. What does upset me is the obscenity of this disease, which cuts one off from friends and family, and really is a death in life. The medicos can offer no treatment but equally they're not prepared to help one opt out of life with at least a little dignity.

Jack, as others, is of course placing his diagnosis in the context of both what he views a 'normal' (in his case biblical) lifespan to be, and also – just as important – is making a judgement about what life itself actually is, and of which he deems social contact and discourse to be an immutable part. His judgements about the role of doctors involve them operating within his personal vision of what it is to be alive, a point we shall return to in later chapters. However, Jack's observation about the treatability of MND/ALS is not without challenge. Bradley argues that:

> It is important that we [neurologists] plant the idea that although the disease may not be curable, it is almost certainly treatable.
>
> (1994: 25)

Norris, one of the pioneers of enhanced medical care for people with MND/ALS, makes a similar point (1994: 30). However it is plain that Jack has fused the ideas of cure and treatment so that they have become co-terminus – it doesn't make sense to him that a disease can be treated but not cured. On the other hand, it is the case that both Bradley and Norris are discussing what they would variously describe as symptomatic or palliative treatments, which may assist in the management (treatment) of symptoms, but do not affect the underlying course of the disease. Thus, the use of the word 'treatment' can be seen both as an annoying fiction to patients, which seems to fudge the terminal time-limited nature of the condition, but still be an established fact to physicians.

Despite the observations above about the complex nature of time in relation to MND/ALS of which chronological time is only a part, there is what might be described as a highly competitive chronological environment in relation to people with the disease. As the mortality curve is so steep in the first few years after diagnosis for the majority of those with MND/ALS, survivors are both statistically highly unusual, and constitute important beacons of hope for those following this difficult path. Of course, there has been a concerted medical attempt to ascertain why some people survive so long and others do not. Scientifically, life expectancy is shorter when:

> initial symptoms involve respiratory or bulbar muscles ... and when patients are older ... in contrast the younger the patient, the longer the life expectancy. When the disease involves exclusively upper motor neurones ... prognosis is much better ... [as it is] in the case of pure lower motor neurone disease.
>
> (Mitsumoto 1994: 15)

However, such descriptions say nothing about the person with the disease – their lives, their determination, their commitments, their ideas, their actions, or who they are. For people with motor neurone disease, it is not so much the nature of the disease as the nature of the person which is important. In this respect, those who survive are not so much considered by other people with the disease to have done so because of some particular pathological or demographic factor, but because of something distinctive about who they are as persons. By postponing death through who they are or what they have done, they can be considered in a sense both to have solved the riddle of existential uncertainty and, in a factual way, to have apparently cheated the normal imperatives of bodily decline through the disease.

By far the most important figure in this respect has become Stephen Hawking, whom we have already noted has achieved a legendary status amongst almost all people with MND/ALS, which cannot be overestimated. Although there are occasional muted scientific questions raised about the diagnostic status of his MND/ALS – for his longevity itself does not fit at all into the 'typical' case of the disease – he has an absolutely unique standing as a person whose apparently transcendent mind is in his body, but somehow not of it. His image amongst others is one in which the bodily ravages of the disease can still be reconciled with a productive – indeed an increasingly productive – life, for the downwards trajectory of the disease is overtaken by the upwards trajectory of the person.

None the less, there are serious concerns about how such images might be deployed when the 'typical' case of MND/ALS appears to be so far removed from that of Stephen Hawking. For Norris, there is even a danger that such images will affect the physician, who, for other reasons as well, may seek to offer a more benign diagnosis than the classical form of MND/ALS which they believe may be present. Such a decision then rebounds when the progression of the disease is far more rapid than the benign diagnosis would warrant (1994: 31).

However the value of transcendent images for people with MND/ALS, no matter what the actual progression of the disease, appears to be underestimated by physicians, who are often most concerned that the patient and their carer should have a 'realistic' view of their physical situation and not fall prey to 'false hopes'.

However, as Murphy describes in relation to a different condition, but which could equally apply to someone with MND/ALS, when:

> the thinking activity of the brain cannot be dissolved into motion, and the mind can no longer be lost in an internal dialogue with physical movement . . . my thoughts and sense of being alive have now driven me back into my brain.
>
> (1987: 102)

The paradox is that the more the physical demands and, in a practical sense, the real effects of MND/ALS take hold, the more likely it is that the escape to hope is contained in a recourse to precisely those images which others may see as being in complete disjunction with the present and immediate future of 'their patient'. We have already considered how such a process may operate in relation to those with malignant brain tumours in Chapter 2 whose multiple strategies for managing the everyday problems of their condition involve retranslating and reinterpreting their worlds in a generally positive way (Salander *et al.* 1996).

In MND/ALS such a process may be more difficult, and positively appropriating what McDonald (1994) rather cumbersomely describes as the psychosocial–spiritual dimensions of the disease made particularly problematic. In this respect, vesting considerable hope in a chronological reprieve, however unrealistic that may appear in particular individual cases, is a personally supportive strategy, which is widely evident in the accounts on which this analysis is based. To announce that one is still here – is alive – after two, three, four, five or ten years, and has exceeded one's personal goal, has 'confounded the doctors', and has proved to be an exception (maybe *the* exception) to the known patterns of the disease, is a considerable achievement. It is an achievement beyond chronology, for it is an achievement in many other dimensions of time as well. It is, moreover, an achievement not only for oneself and one's family, but also an achievement for all people with MND/ALS. For if even only one individual surpasses the 'normal' or 'typical' expectations of chronological life after diagnosis, it both casts doubt on major elements of that typicality and provides hope for others to continue the struggle to try and 'beat the disease'. In this respect, not only do individual accounts, such as that of Neil below, announce the survival of another person, but also the increasingly important electronic media for people with MND/ALS, such as the ALSIG (ALS Interest Group) Newsletter available through the Internet (the

World Wide Web), which broadcasts such information to a wider and appreciative audience:

> The most important thing is that I am still alive. The doctor gave me not more than two years to live, and here I am, it's now five years since he told me. Things are hard but I am still struggling against it [the MND/ALS].

In practice, of course, despite the firm (scientifically based) knowledge of doctors and other health-care staff that the outcome of the disease is almost entirely predictable in the vast majority of cases, and their concern that patients do not have an inappropriately positive view of their condition, those concerned directly, personally and continuously with the health care of people with MND/ALS also sometimes conspire in a gentle way to encourage the thought that disease 'burn out' may occur in individual cases (Norris 1994: 39–40), or generate hope by indicating that:

> some patients will have five, fifteen or even more years ahead of them, and perhaps even outlive the practitioner.
>
> (McDonald 1994: 226)

Whilst the proportion of such patients is relatively low, such an approach is not only understandable, it is often unavoidable for those in day-to-day contact with people with MND/ALS and their relatives, as the cold light of scientific knowledge is placed in the context of the range of possibilities which might conceivably occur, as well as in the context of the management of sensitive interpersonal relationships.

LOOKING FORWARD AND LOOKING BACK: THE PERSONAL AND SOCIAL CONTEXT OF MND/ALS IN LATE MIDDLE AGE

Formally and statistically the most frequent first expressions and recognition of what turn out to be the symptoms of motor neurone disease occur at one of the key contemporary transitional points in life between 55 and 70 years old. Between these ages a wide range of often interlinked and major changes occur in the personal, social and economic framework of individuals' worlds, in which for an increasing constituency, as Peter Laslett anticipates, the attractions of the 'Third Age' beyond retirement are welcomed with hope rather than with fear. It is just at this point, it seems to many, that MND/ALS strikes.

In explaining the particular potency of the diagnosis of MND/ALS, and how destructive it appears to be for those who are touched by it at these ages, we must consider the profound association between personal expectations and such a social context. As John indicated, looking back on this transition (for him) to retirement, in which MND/ALS had robustly intervened:

> We [he and his wife] were looking forward so much to what we could do when I retired from my job. Gill [his wife] had put up with so much, what with so many moves; my overseas postings, as well as working all hours, so I really owed this retirement to her. We had planned to do so many things together, and had already worked out exactly how we would spend our time, and then this happened [the symptoms and then the diagnosis of MND/ALS]. It's taken our future away, Gill is so bitter about it, and so am I. She's sacrificed so much already, but for what?

In many respects, it is as though the onset of the disease has catapulted John from an active working life one moment, to the immediate contemplation of decline and death. In effect, he has missed a life-stage. A very significant life-stage which would have completed for him a socially and morally appropriate life trajectory. He had paid his dues to work (and society), and more particularly his wife had done so through valiantly supporting him, and now they had been cheated out of what they both felt they deserved – indeed what society 'owed' them.

John's situation raises a number of broader issues into which the onset of MND/ALS must be contextualised. In Chapter 1 we noted a demographic paradox associated with the major increase in life expectancy in industrialised societies and a corresponding increase in the incidence of the disease. On the one hand, populations as a whole are living longer; on the other hand, they are now falling prey to conditions to which a shorter life span would not have left them liable. In John's case, as in many others with the onset of MND/ALS, the enticing prospect of an even longer life well into old age has itself been circumscribed by a condition about which in earlier generations little was known – not because it was seriously under diagnosed, but because few people would have reached the age at which it was generally expressed and experienced.

Now, most personal and social futures are built on an assumed symmetry of life stages in which lengthy periods of childhood/full-time education, and paid working life, are implicitly balanced by an anticipated lengthy – and relatively active – period of later life. In considering the microcosm of John's world, as well as in considering the larger, even global, framework within which the issue is often debated, 'being old' or entering 'old age' is a relative concept – indeed a social construction. For example, in a comparison between the views of 16 to 24-year-olds, and those aged 75, a survey for Age Concern (1992) indicated that whereas for the former the mean age at which old age began was sixty-three, for the latter it began at seventy-six. Thus, the perception of being old is considered by many, particularly chronologically older people themselves, to be entirely related to their present age and situation. For John, being older was just one contextualised component of a life-course, rather than being in the definitive, discrete category 'old age'. He is not entering 'old age' as the end of his life at 65; he is (or was) entering another more positive phase – in many respects the beginning of a new life. Manton and Stallard (1991) suggest that for most late-middle-aged people this is a realistic prospect. Life expectancy for those who reach the age of sixty-five is approximately 14 years for men, and 18 years for women, of which 12 and 13.6 years respectively will be what Manton and Stallard describe as 'active', in which there will no major functional impediments to everyday living.

There is an additional problematic component to what is almost always a very truncated life span with MND/ALS for people such as John, and that is the loss of anticipated freedom in retirement, before the life itself is lost. Although personal, social and financial freedom, autonomy and choice are often considered to be vested almost exclusively in younger people, studies are increasingly indicating that it is the freedom that older people feel they enjoy which allows them, in general, to have such a positive attitude to their situation. For example, in a survey for British Gas (1991) in response to the question, 'As you grow older will you enjoy life less, the same or more than you used to do?', of those aged 55–74 only 27 per cent said less, and of those aged 75 and over only 38 per cent said less. The single most important reason for enjoying life was the freedom they had (83 per cent). Despite concerns about financial constraints, for many on the verge of retirement being free of daily (paid) work commitments – if they were able to – as well as free of many of the more burdensome duties associated with a full-time working life were all things to which to look forward.

There is also another set of general demographic and social features which make the onset of MND/ALS so poignant for couples at this pre-retirement/immediate post-retirement age. In addition to an increasingly nucleated family structure in which more and more activities, interests and interactions centre around a small family unit (especially the married or partnered couple), women tend to marry older men, and differential life expectancy means that many more of those women are likely to be widowed. The effects of these processes in Britain are quite striking, in 1985 at 65 or older 78 per cent of all males were married compared to 46 per cent of females, whilst in the same age range 50 per cent of women and 18 per cent of men were widowed (British Gas Report 1991: 23). Thus although it is (statistically) likely that women will enter into widowhood as they reach older ages, the advent of MND/ALS is likely to substantially increase this possibility at an earlier age, as well as leaving those women with a very changed set of social circumstances, and almost certainly a changed set of financial circumstances as well. As Slater puts it:

> Later life is a woman's issue because there are many more women to experience it, and relatively more so at increasing ages.
>
> (1995: 35)

These, and other far more personal issues, are precisely why women, especially as wives, partners and carers, are so locked in to the pressures and problems which MND/ALS, as a terminal diagnosis brings, in late middle age.

THE CONTEXT OF DIAGNOSIS IN THE OLDER OLD

Although it is argued, and far more frequently now, that being old is not a disease, or is in itself a medical condition, in practice the relatively linear statistical association of what are usually described as chronic diseases with increasing age (especially rheumatoid arthritis, heart and vascular conditions, and problems with the senses, such as hearing and eyesight) tends to undermine these claims – at least in terms of everyday assumptions and discourse. Even when research-based data suggest that despite the presence of these conditions many older people are functionally relatively competent – indeed in many senses remarkably so given their catalogue of (in medical terms) increasing bodily impairments – a healthy old age still seems often to be rather a surprise.

Thus, at the oldest older ages the kinds of symptoms that MND/ALS presents may well fit almost easily at first into the daily vagaries which attend the normal course of living. It is indeed this factor which has been used to explain not only why the initial recognition of the seriousness of the symptoms of MND/ALS may be delayed by those who prove to have the disease, but also why physicians may have failed to recognise the condition in the past, thus leading to an 'artifactual' rather than a 'real' increase in the numbers of those with MND/ALS. Although such a claim appears plausible and fits well with other studies which identify changing practices as well as changing disease categories for major shifts in the prevalence (and incidence) of diseases, there are good grounds for suggesting that, in the case of MND/ALS, such an explanation is only likely to encompass a modest component of the changing distribution of MND/ALS.

Explaining directly and immediately what the relatively unmitigated consequences of the disease might mean to the older person and their family, when both the latters' agendas are fixed on relatively benign remaining years, may produce an extended and very problematic dialogue for the doctor, dealing as much with difficult extra, as well as intra-medical factors. Given that the course of the disease is generally swifter in older people; that some of the more problematic stages of the disease may be compressed together, and that the process of dying in itself is, for all, an unknown process, it may be deemed not only kinder but 'more responsible' not to reveal the condition in all its future starkness. Indeed, if family members become aware at an early stage of the prognosis of MND/ALS, whether by default or by design, they may feel compelled to assist a doctor in such a strategy, for if they do not, in addition to confronting the 'ordinary' functional problems of the oldest old in a very exaggerated form, they are immediately faced with possibly irresolvable discussions on a wide range of painful moral questions – for example, about the 'fairness of life', and the meaning of 'good' and 'bad' deaths. However as we argue in Chapter 6, the familial impact of MND/ALS is usually such that, whether or not the very oldest person is aware of the diagnosis, family members heavily involved in the care and support of the person with MND/ALS feel that they have experienced both life and death in its rawest form.

There is of course a particular irony in relation to the onset of MND/ALS at older ages for, as we note at various points throughout this book, the disease which has come to represent 'old age' at its most problematic is not MND/ALS but Alzheimer's Disease, or in a more generic form dementia. Statistically this view is understandable as there is a clear linear increase in the prevalence of dementia with increasing age. As Black *et al.* (1991: 88) show from their review of many studies mean prevalence rates of dementia were 5.7 per cent at ages 75–79, 10.5 per cent at ages 80–85, and rising to 39 per cent in the tenth decade of life. From their earlier review Korten *et al.* (1997) conclude that the prevalence of dementia increases exponentially with age, doubling every 5.1 years. Perhaps surprisingly there is little evidence – apart from a small number of individual cases – that people with MND/ALS, however old they may be, also have dementia, even though they are likely to show the normal modest cognitive deficits of ageing persons (Korten *et al.* 1997). Thus older people with MND/ALS can be considered to be almost a physical mirror image of those with damaged cognitive and other mental processes in dementia. In brief people with MND/ALS are often faced with autonomous choice without the possibility of commensurate physical action, whereas people with dementia may be faced with physical action without the possibility – at least according to others – of autonomous choice.

However, the world of older people is of course a complex one, as we have indicated earlier in this chapter, not only because of the physical vagaries and problems which may afflict them more than others, but because of other – usually younger people's – perceptions of their competence. Even if older people with MND/ALS do not have the same reported prevalence of dementia as other old people, they may still, through a combination of their MND/ALS and their age, exhibit traits and behaviours which are considered by others to render them 'typical' old people, of which the most 'typical' signs are cognitive impairment (dementia), mobility problems and incontinence (Mitteness and Barker 1995). Although incontinence is a relatively rare complication of MND/ALS itself (Norris 1994: 34–5), there tends to be a compressing of categories in social judgements about older people in which it is assumed that one of these three signs is unlikely to occur without the others. Bill, an articulate eighty-year-old with MND/ALS, expresses some of his frustrations:

> The problem I face with this dreadful disease is not only how quickly I am going downhill, but I can only just shuffle about, and now I'm having big difficulties letting people know what I want. Before I got the MND/ALS I prided myself on how I was, people used to say 'He's sprightly for his age!' Now everyone treats me as stupid, and I've become just another stupid old man to them who doesn't know what he wants, and can't do anything anyway.

However, for other older old people the MND/ALS does result, in effect, in an accelerated decline of their already depleted physical powers and is seen by their relatives as very concerning, but is perceived none the less in the context of a situation when arrangements were already being made for their longer-term care. In such cases, the major issue is how to incorporate the additional practical burdens of MND/ALS, but through a prism where their future decline and death are implicitly part of an unspoken family agenda. This is clearly not the situation with younger people diagnosed with MND/ALS.

YOUNG ADULTS AND MND/ALS: THE TRAGEDY OF A DISEASE OUT OF TIME

Although those over fifty are the predominant age group by far who are diagnosed with MND/ALS, the personal and social resonance of a diagnosis at a younger age is very powerful. Bradley expresses a doctor's eye view of the relationship he sees between diagnosis at an older and at a younger age:

> In a frail eighty-year-old, the diagnosis is not such a burden to the doctor, but in the all-too-frequent patient in their twenties or thirties with a young family and so much life before him or her, ALS [MND] is a tragedy.

(1994: 27)

In fact, as we noted in Chapter 1, not only is the proportion of those diagnosed with MND/ALS under fifty decreasing with some rapidity, but their absolute numbers are declining as well. However, as Bradley implies, the key issue is not so much the number (absolute or relative) of those in the younger age groups diagnosed with

MND/ALS, but the personal and social loss incurred by such a diagnosis. Bradley is broadly concurring with Jack's idea earlier in this chapter that there is an appropriate age to live and an appropriate age to die, in which the tragedy of death is inversely related to the length of life.

In practice what might be regarded as the technical issues of the management of a declining body are not dissimilar in older or younger people with MND/ALS, for the ways in which the destruction of motor neurones affects bodily function, and in particular muscular control, are also similar. However, in addition to the likelihood that younger people will live longer with MND/ALS, and that their respective physical trajectories will be more varied, what is extraordinarily different, is the personal and social repercussions of such a diagnosis. These repercussions in their turn affect how technical tasks are perceived and organised, and in particular how those involved professionally understand and manage their role. Bradley's comments above suggest how difficult it is – we would say impossible – to separate out the pathology of the disease from the nature and characteristics of the social person. In his comments he is going well beyond terse descriptions of the demographic profile of people with MND/ALS to make a social – and personal – judgement about younger people and MND/ALS.

Certainly it would be difficult in personal, social and cultural terms, whatever the similarities of the pathology of the disease between older and younger people, to be other than particularly struck by the immediate dilemmas which faced Geoff and his young family, in what many might describe as the 'prime of their lives':

I was 38 years at the time I found out I had MND . . . married with three children, 8 years, 4 years and a new baby 6 months old, who I thought I would never see grow up, and he would hardly ever remember me. My wife would be widowed, and being self-employed, where would the money to support them come from? I was going to die before my parents and it worried me as to how they would cope with the situation – [but] I did not worry for myself at all. I had had a good and full life up to that time, with no regrets. Everything in my life had gone very smoothly . . . [However] all my doctor said to me [at the time of the diagnosis] was to give up work and enjoy myself as much as I could for my remaining months/years. I felt terribly isolated then and it was only the marvellous support of my family which saw me through this difficult period . . . I have been one of the lucky patients as the disease has progressed very slowly, and I am still able to carry on a normal way of life. Ten years on my family obviously means everything to me.

However, there is a social danger in characterising Geoff's case as representing, and being representative of the essence of the dilemmas of all people with MND/ALS. For whilst there are core personal and social values which Geoff's case confronts in a direct, and one might say heart-rending way, the particularly difficult situation of the many more older people with MND/ALS may be relatively neglected in such a focus. None the less, of course, the resonance of the tragedy of younger people with serious, or terminal illness, whether it be MND/ALS or not, is such that it is difficult to set aside when his – and his family's – future now seems to be in the past.

Geoff's case, and other similar cases, do raise other specific questions, about both the role of individual factors in the genesis of MND/ALS, as well as questions about how people cope with what are commonly described as the psychosocial dimensions of the disease.

UNDERSTANDING, COPING AND MANAGING: INDIVIDUAL FACTORS AND MND/ALS

In a disease such as MND/ALS, the issue of the relative longevity of individuals, as well as the ways in which they may personally manage their particular circumstances, prompts questions about the relationship of their personality, attitudes and approaches to the condition. In common with other serious or terminal conditions there have been attempts to ascertain whether there is a particular personality profile which characterises people with disease.

Three studies, all undertaken in the United States have, overall, produced inconclusive results in this respect. Although a small study by Brown and Mueller (1970) comparing ten people with ALS/MND, with ten who had inoperable cancer, concluded that the former demonstrated a significantly greater perception of being in control of lives, and what they described as a lifetime pattern of active mastery, these findings were not endorsed in a larger study of forty patients (Houpt *et al.* 1977). In a later study using the MMPI

(Minnesota MultiPhasic Inventory) comparing patients with ALS/MND with a general medical population, thirty-eight out of forty-four of the patients did not differ from that population (Peters *et al.* 1978). Following these studies, there has been little scientific energy directed towards further general studies of the personalities of people with MND/ALS. Greater attention has however increasingly been paid to investigating the psychological context and consequences of the disease. In particular, concern has been directed to the general affective status of people with MND/ALS, and to what extent their profile differs from or is similar to that of equivalent general populations. In addition, the basis on which individual patients cope with the disease has been the subject of examination, and whether there are certain key attitudinal or other factors which determine, or at least are strongly associated with, effective coping. In relation to a general affective profile of people with MND/ALS, McDonald summarises her conclusions as follows:

> [Our] evaluation [of 144 ALS/MND patients] included tests that measured depression, hopelessness, perceived stress, anger expression, loneliness, health locus of control, life satisfaction and purpose in life. Surprisingly, patients' scores for each test scale covered a broad range, suggesting great variability in psychosocial-spiritual status. When the average scores for these test were compared to those of a normal, healthy population, the only differences were that the ALS [MND] patients exhibited more depression . . . and had a more external locus of control. [However] neither depression nor an external locus of control is unusual in patients with chronic disease. The wide variability and overall normality of these results suggest that there is no predictable psychosocial-spiritual profile for the ALS [MND] patient.
>
> (1994: 207)

Furthermore, as McDonald indicates, and has been found in two British studies (Hunter *et al.* 1993; Hogg *et al.* 1994), even with a relatively wide range of psychological measures, psychosocial (or in McDonald's terms, psychosocial-spiritual) status has a very complex relationship to other proxy measures of disease progression. Factors such as age, length of illness, mode of onset, functional status, measures of the severity of the disease, and even dependence on a ventilator do not in any striking sense differentiate patients into very clear psychosocial categories (McDonald 1994: 208; Hunter *et al.* 1993). To put the point in a more emphatic way, there is no direct or linear correlation between the state of the disease and the state of the person. Indeed, reported oddly but succinctly, in some cases the disease was worse but the person felt better. These observations raise interesting and important issues as to why this apparent lack of a clear congruence between psychosocial and disease-based factors should be present.

A scientifically plausible argument in circumstances such as this is that the instruments used to measure psychosocial status are not sufficiently sensitive to detect a phenomenon – increasing psychosocial distress – which is probably there but too elusive to capture at present, or those existing instruments have been deployed inappropriately or incorrectly. However, in the case of all three of the studies mentioned above, the instruments used were well validated and have been regularly used to detect various components of psychosocial distress in other conditions. A more feasible explanation is one which McDonald herself suggests; that is:

> Many factors influence where a patient will fall on the psychosocial-spiritual spectrum, including physical parameters associated with the progression of the disease, social factors, the patient's environment and family relationships, the patient's spirit, and the patient's experience with the health care system.
>
> (1994: 208)

Given the reach of scientific method, most of these elements, and others, could in principle be measurable, but it might be argued that the particular conjunction of them operating in any particular individual's life, as they continually engage in a struggle to make sense of their situation, is not likely to be easily amenable to precise scientific analysis. Furthermore, even if they were, such a process would still not be able to engage with the person's existential quest for the management of meaning in their lives, for the reasons we elucidated at the outset of this chapter.

Another approach which is widely used in practice to categorise and make sense of patient's psychosocial status in MND/ALS by professional caregivers, is through deploying an adaptive model. Such a model, which usually includes the elements of shock, denial, anger, depression, acknowledgement and acceptance, is often assumed to operate in a sequenced linear order, in which the general goal of the health care giver is to facilitate the accomplishment of the various stages in order to enable the patient to accept their situation. However, in addition to the evidence for the existence of such a staged process being problematic, professional caregivers may find that they are operating with categories which themselves have multiple meanings for both their patients and themselves. In the case of 'denial' for example, it can either be considered to be an unhelpful category to get 'stuck in', or:

> a protective coping mechanism that helps a person who has received a terminal diagnosis retain psychological equilibrium.
>
> (ALS Society of Canada 1994: 9)

Although there are indeed major conceptual problems linked with what 'denial' might be, as well as with its position in the patient's armoury of techniques for the management of their MND/ALS, in principle the same argument can be developed in relation to the other staged categories. In the end, as McDonald indicates, 'each patient and their spouse is unique' (1994: 222) and thus the use of a template of staged responses to the onset and course of the disease to place upon the person with MND/ALS may not be a profitable exercise – certainly from that person's point of view in meeting the everyday challenges of the disease.

Chapter 4

Everyday life in the early stages of motor neurone disease

BODIES, MINDS AND BRAINS: UNDERSTANDING THE SOCIAL FRAMEWORK OF COMMUNICATION IN MND/ALS

The varied catalogue of possible signs and symptoms of MND/ALS which we outlined in Chapter 1 ensures that, whatever the particular course of the disease, life with the condition is a demanding exercise – even from its onset. This is so, not only in ensuring that the complex array of problems stemming from the lessening in muscular control as well as muscular debilitation is technically redressed and assisted as much as possible. In managing, for most people with the disease, it is also a relatively relentless decline in key body systems and everyday performance, which focuses attention at the same time on the past (i.e. what has been lost), the present (what remains), and on the future (what else is there to lose?). Keiran reflects on the workings of his body after the onset of MND/ALS:

I am still active physically and mentally; only my speech and swallowing are affected substantially by MND though the grip of my left hand is going and the right one is showing some signs of deterioration. There are occasional creaks, cramps and tremors all over the place. I do my swallowing and speech exercises but there seems to be a slow but irregular decline since July when the diagnosis was made and since the middle of last year when minor symptoms obviously appeared. I am conscious of these changes though whether this is more or less than normal I do not know. [All this is in the context of the fact] that I have hardly been ill for 50 years and only had one potentially dangerous illness in my life, a mild attack of diphtheria at the age of 9. Does this make one more or less twitchy about the state of one's body?

There is always a concern about the next bodily symptom to show itself, as Henry notes:

In the past month one other symptom has occurred. It is a pain in the upper right arm muscle like one might expect from sawing logs or bowling at cricket. It is worse when I lift anything even a cup of tea and is relieved when I hold it with my left hand and is worse when I try to turn in bed.

Joy lists the ways in which she believes her body, or rather 'the body' – as it has now become an object to her – reflects her diagnosis of MND/ALS:

1 The loss of feeling in the feet.
2 The stubbing and falls.
3 The lack of grip of hands.
4 The spasmodic severe tingling in extremities.
5 The giddiness and general unsteadiness.
6 The swaying when the eyes are closed.
7 The reverse reaction of the toes when bottom of feet scraped.
8 The husky voice and loss of voice when lungs, vocal chords etc. are down.
9 The flopping and dropping of feet.
10 The loss of control following shingles.
11 The awkward hand control of small objects.
12 The continuous pain in muscle upper right arm.
13 The symptoms found in a middle/old age person.

Such a set of difficulties invariably raise a wider range of issues about the relationship between yourself and your body, in which who 'you are' may be at the core, especially if body skills, bodily performance, and bodily presentation to others have been a significant feature of life before MND/ALS – as they will have been in greater or lesser degree to everyone. In addition, as in Keiran's case, a long-lasting pride in previously maintaining a healthy body has clearly conditioned his own views about his body and himself.

For most people with the disease, and certainly for many doctors diagnosing and offering management to them, their brains are considered cognitively 'normal'. But there is a conceptual difficulty in where the problem lies if the mind (the self) is normal, and the muscles in the body are – or would be – normal given appropriate control and regular exercise, and the brain is also normal. It appears that this conceptual difficulty is solved by considering the problem to lie in communicative processes between the mind and the body but outside the brain, somewhere in the nervous system. The disease, in this sense, is in the body, but not of the body; although, at the same time, this perspective leaves the brain, and mind, relatively untouched as a source of trouble. In the everyday management of MND/ALS, especially in the earlier stages of the disease, such a view is helpful in working through the various processes of deterioration brought about by the presence of the disease – for indeed the focus is on enhancing communication both within the body, and between self and others. However, as we shall discuss later, this perspective leads to considerable difficulty and confusion in considering the terminal stages of the disease.

The emphasis on the significance of increasingly ineffective communicative processes from the brain to the body, immediately reorientates attention on everyday issues of time and bodily performance, which is where we began this brief discussion. In this respect, the difficulty of messages 'getting through' to muscles because of the destruction of motor neurones is helpfully considered in the context of Slater's information processing metaphor:

> the train might arrive late at its destination because it travelled the route more slowly, or because it was diverted onto a route which was more circuitous.
>
> (1995: 62)

Although Slater is discussing the effect of cognitive deficits on information processing, extending the metaphor the problem for people with MND/ALS is that over time and in due course the train may never arrive, because it cannot travel at all by any route, all those routes are destroyed.

The slowing down, and eventual destruction of the possibility of internal body communications through key aspects of the central nervous system, produces a paradox. On the one hand, time seems to stand still for tasks that were routinely and quickly undertaken only a few weeks or few days ago, and which now 'take forever' to accomplish. On the other hand, time has speeded up as the consecutive loss of physical skills accelerates – often, it appears, exponentially. A combination of these two apparently contradictory factors, time apparently standing virtually still on the one hand, so that 'nothing' is accomplished, and accelerating on the other hand so that far more needs to be accomplished, creates a difficult environment in which to undertake the increasingly complex but necessary routine domestic tasks of personal care, eating and drinking, as well as developing increasingly novel ways of effective communication with others. At an earlier stage of the disease, Greg thinks in increasing detail about time and the relationship of some of his symptoms to his diagnosis:

It is now some three months since the MND but there has been very little change to confirm or to challenge it. Walking is gradually becoming more tiring but that could be aging or natural circulation factors. The only symptom which seems to be more pronounced is the aching of the muscle in the upper right arm . . . which is now more or less continuous and severe at times, making turning in bed at night really painful. I am not certain but believe it wakes me about 2am after going to bed at 10pm. If it is not responsible then some other factor is now regularly causing me to wake. Up to say four months ago I always slept through to about 6 to 6.30am I am due to see my doctor for a 3 monthly check up at the end of June, at which I will discuss this.

In some respects, although what we have described as the technical management of a wide range of declining physical skills is indeed a difficult process to manage, it brings with it other potent reminders of the changing world of the person with MND/ALS. Even if MND/ALS seems to gnaw away at what may appear to be basic functional competencies, the salience of each of these competencies in relation to each other is bound up with how others see us – in relation to what they think makes us the individual we are, as well as how we fit into broader categories such as being old or young, male or female, and so on. Of course, with the advent of very serious illness our social world generally changes, and often quite rapidly. Thus, people with MND/ALS are brought into contact with a greater number of people from the world of the sick – that is, other people who are themselves ill or those who care for them – and their contact with others who are 'healthy' tends to be reduced. In this process, the instrumental and expressive components of relationships with others centre more and more on the issues which surround the declining body and its consequences, or at the very least it takes increasing effort to turn both behaviours and beliefs to other issues. Reconstructing sets of relationships with other people around the demands of managing MND/ALS leads to a difficult set of tasks, none more so than finding and establishing effective contact with expert health professionals, and integrating their skills with those of the person with MND/ALS and their family.

BUILDING EXPERTISE IN THE EVERYDAY MANAGEMENT OF MND/ALS: PEOPLE WITH MND/ALS, THEIR FAMILIES AND PROFESSIONAL SUPPORT

It would be hard to find another disease which simultaneously taxed so many aspects of any formal health care system, and the work of those within it. We have already noted a number of these points that relate to such a system's capacity, as well as that of those within it, to shift from a curative to a symptomatic treatment or palliative role; the ability to work effectively with major health problems with older people; the ability to confront and manage issues of dying and death on a continuous basis; the ability to operate both within scientific knowledge, but beyond it at the same time; the ability to synthesise and develop fruitful and deep collaborative relationships between radically different professional perspectives and techniques; the ability to acknowledge, and largely work within the personal perspectives of individuals and families, whilst understanding that such perspectives within families may differ, and contradict each other; and finally to be able to apply the broad technical skills, usually learnt through a single professional education, to the complexities of each individual with the disease.

A further complication for many health care staff, especially those at a local community level, who become involved with people with MND/ALS is that they are often meeting people in that position for the first time, as indeed may be their managers, or senior colleagues. In this respect, the learning curve for all those involved is sharp and substantial, and problematic. No one, at that stage, may be an expert whose knowledge base is specifically targeted on the condition – even those staff whose rationale and existence is based on their special claim to expertise in health care. Indeed, all may be seeking expertise from each other as the person with MND/ALS and their relatives seek urgent information from health care staff about current practical issues, as well as the course and future problems associated with the disease. Similarly, those health care staff are themselves engaged in learning from the 'lived expertise' of people with the condition.

The experiences of Edward, in relation to his wife, highlight the difficulties of the process of finding expert assistance in the face of a number of additional problems:

[After being given the diagnosis by the neurologist] her muscular deterioration . . . continued. Later that month, weakness in her legs caused her to fracture her ankle . . . at no time did the local GP link this with the MND. In fact, after the fracture, I took her to the local hospital six miles away and it was expertly set and plastered. There was no reference to her medical condition whatsoever. On a subsequent visit to the GP the diagnosis of the neurologist at the previous clinical appointment was corroborated in a letter which the GP read out to my wife and I. Even at this stage, the GP indicated that he knew little about the disease. Muscular deterioration in both legs was now apparent. Again no advice was forthcoming. I have to admit, that my wife did not want to know and this inhibited me from getting a second opinion although the GP had offered this facility. Another local GP meeting her socially offered to put her in touch with two other local [MND/ALS] sufferers. This she declined. A little later, when my wife was now wheelchair bound and totally dependent on me, I requested physiotherapy help from my local GP. After an inordinate amount of time and several reminders a very helpful physiotherapist . . . appeared. She indicated that she could only visit the local health centre once a week and that my wife would have to be given her physiotherapy there. On her observation of the physiotherapy I was giving my wife, she suggested that this was even more than she could give. After a big battle I found that I could join a group at a local hospital which organised 'hydrotherapy', to stimulate circulation . . . We joined and this gave my wife a tremendous boost to her morale, since it allowed her body to function in ways which she thought she had lost. Could this not have been done initially?

There are several key issues in Edward's case which form a common thread through many other accounts of people with MND/ALS, and their families. The first is the ignorance of the GP about the specific features of MND/ALS, and particularly about how Edward's wife might be supported by him (the GP) or other health care professionals – although he did attempt to assist in other ways. The second is the relatively terse and cursory relationship between specialist care (in hospital) and primary care (the GP) – in which the specialist hospital's role appears to have begun and ended, as in so many other cases, with the confirmation of the diagnosis. The third is what often appears in the accounts of people with MND/ALS as an endemic problem from their point of view which is the difficulty of receiving continuing and appropriate physiotherapy support, which is a part of the larger battle to marshall formal health care resources in such a situation. The fourth is the extent to which not only Edward's time, but also his own considerable expertise, is now involved in the care of his wife.

On a broader issue, the balance between professionally based formal health care and informal health care by self, family and friends, Edward's position echoes that of not only many other people with MND/ALS, but also people with a wide range of other conditions. In addition, in common with many families with MND/ALS in their midst, Edward is managing his wife's condition at home. As Tennstadt and McKinlay note in their study of informal care for older people, the dominant constituency of those with MND/ALS:

> The data show that older people receive most of their assistance from family and friends. Further, of those receiving help from both informal and formal sources, most of the care is received informally. In addition . . . the amount of informal care is substantially higher than the amount of formal services for [older people] . . . who are severely impaired. Therefore, contrary to assumptions, even when greater needs necessitate more help, informal caregivers provide greater amounts of assistance when compared with utilisation of formal services. And in those areas of help where one might expect some shift towards formal services because services are well established and readily available . . . the data reveal large amounts of informal help associated with larger amounts of formal services, again with the former exceeding the latter. It is *not* [author's emphasis] the case that informal care complements, or is ancillary to, formal services. Rather formal services complement or are ancillary to, a well established, pervasive, and continuing informal system of care.

> (1989: 160)

In discussing the role of formal health care in relation to MND/ALS, it is generally agreed by agencies that:

Health care providers need to form an ongoing partnership with people with [MND/ALS] and their families in order to devise and maintain a care plan that is orientated to the person not the disease.

(ALS Society of Canada 1994: 8)

The availability of such services organised in ways in which there can be an effective intermeshing of informal and formal care is very variable, thus:

the highly specialised types of services needed by the patient are rarely obtained, so the bulk of home care service frequently falls to a relative, friend or other caregiver.

(Parks 1994: 197)

As far as formal health care services are concerned this may always prove to be the case, as Tennstadt and McKinlay imply above, not only for resource reasons – although this is a critical factor – but also because of the particular characteristics of family life at home. As Rubinstein argues, the home may be considered in two parallel ways:

as a setting for the more practical, tactical tasks of caregiving . . . [or] alternatively, home may be defined in terms of a moral function. The home expresses love, unity, and caring and is believed to have a curative or restorative effect above and beyond its technical role in facilitating care.

(1990: 39)

In this process:

Basic to the meaning of home are the various elements of control, security, family development, independence, comfort, protection, feelings and the presence of people . . . [therefore] to keep a sick person at home means, in essence, that the person is not fully 'sick'. In comparison with other alternatives, to be at home represents a more active personhood. The function of the home as protector and familiar, may play an important part in modulating illness.

(1990: 39)

Thus, whilst those involved in the provision of formal care services focus on the importance of technical skills gained from professional training as the main element of home care – for example, Parks, in a continuation of the quotation above, notes that nursing care is crucial as relatives or friends are not 'licensed or skilled in [MND/ALS] care' – family members focus on a combination of what Rubinstein describes as the moral as well as the practical tasks of home care. As we argue in the next section of this chapter, the 'home' aspect of home care is as important as its professionally judged technical proficiency.

The taxing problems of finding and drawing on the wide and usually dispersed range of professional expertise necessary for the management of MND/ALS, have led over the last twenty years to the foundation of voluntary societies in North America and Britain, as well as more recently other countries, not only to support research into the disease, but more importantly – from an immediate point of view – to provide an expert resource for people with MND/ALS and their families. In fact, in the accounts in this analysis, the relevant main voluntary society in England, the MNDA (the Motor Neurone Disease Association) has clearly come to the rescue on many occasions through its advice and support network for those who were faced with apparently intractable difficulties in obtaining support through standard formal health care structures. One of these accounts indicates the background to the foundation of the MNDA. Sally says:

> William wanted to know everything about MND. He had a wife and young children and wanted to be able to plan the rest of his life. Our GP had never had an MND case in 25 years of practice. The hospital were of no help whatsoever, at any time. We were not offered a social worker (presumably because we were seen to be coping OK) until I asked for help . . . then it was too late for my husband, he would have nothing to do with her . . . We had never heard of MND and nobody we knew had heard of it . . . It was obviously a shock to know he had not long to live. He would not let me tell any family or friends because he knew it wouldn't show for a while and he didn't want people looking at him, waiting for him to die . . . [However] gradually we told family and friends after we had come to terms with it ourselves. Everyone was very supportive, but of course, we all had a feeling of helplessness. After William gave up work he wrote to a doctor in America whose article he had read in a library book. He put us in touch with the ALS Society in America and a leading neurologist, [and the latter] put us in touch with the Muscular

Dystrophy Group who told us of a small group of MND patients wishing to form their own group. We contacted them and together formed the MNDA and drew up the Constitution and formed a Committee. This did more for William than any doctors. It kept his mind occupied (which was all he had left) and he knew he was helping future MND sufferers.

Since its foundation, and through a welfare structure organised round Regional Care Advisers, Welfare Officers in a large branch structure, and more recently through supporting a small array of clinical centres, it appears that the MNDA has managed over time to come into contact with many people with MND/ALS and either provide expertise itself, or coordinate other available expertise. A similar 'alternative health service' for MND/ALS organised through voluntary societies has become a key feature of skilled advice about the disease in North America. For Fran, this arrangement clearly worked better than the other possibilities for support and help she had tried previously:

[After my diagnosis following choking attacks] . . . I was perfectly fit in every way but [I was told that] my nerve endings were frayed and weren't delivering messages to the throat muscles, which was the reason for the choking. No name was ever given but I asked if my voice would ever recover and I was told that it was a degenerative disease for which there was no antidote and they could only hope to alleviate the symptoms by trial and error . . . Then I saw my own private doctor and we asked him to fill in our private insurance form. He confessed to us that in all his years in practice, he had never come up against this disease, which did nothing to reassure me . . . it was only when we returned home and looked at the nature of the disease that we met 'Motor Neurone Disease' for the first time . . . [Later] . . . I chanced to see in the newspapers an appeal for funds for the MNDA, whom my husband immediately contacted. I can only say the response was instant and, in no time at all, we had made contact with the speech therapist at the local hospital. It was she who explained . . . the disease [to me] and [told me] that mine was bulbar palsy; she told me that I wouldn't choke to death and taught me to relax in an attack – which gave me greatly needed confidence . . . My voice has completely gone now, as a result of two colds last January, but the MNDA has supplied me with a means of communication, together with a suction pump for dealing with saliva and mucous. We maintain contact with the hospital and the speech therapist but have discontinued visits to the neurologist, which were totally non-productive.

There are several difficulties outlined in these and similar accounts which are partly concerned with ensuring that information is coincident with that requested and required by people with the condition and their relatives at the beginning of the disease. They are also partly concerned with determining where the necessary array of expertise for managing the condition is available, and how that expertise can be obtained. However, often the key issue is not so much either of these issues, but is concerned with the flow of information and expertise in relation to the trajectory of the condition.

In a progressive condition such as MND/ALS, the rapidity with which everyday problems can accumulate and compound each other is such that the usual pace at which community-based health care provision operates can be quickly and frustratingly overtaken and outdistanced. Many accounts contain examples of advice, expertise or equipment which was urgently needed at one particular time, and which may have been laboriously engineered through formal health care procedures, but that only materialise at a point where they are completely redundant. In such cases, as in many others which arise during the disease, people with MND/ALS, or their relatives, develop their own solutions as best they can to those difficulties, as we discuss in the next section of this chapter. In Adrienne's case, she finally learnt how to seek what she needed for her husband, but in the face of a great deal of frustration:

> What is really needed . . . is the practical help we finally got. We just did not realise what help could be obtained [even equipment] all on loan too. Just [to have] a phone number when in need, or feeling very low is important, then one can cope. With broken nights when sleep is lacking, the mind is too tired to see what help you need to ask for. And that is the trouble, you have to know what to ask for, and who to ask for it. Often we learned this too late to help. We felt that the consultant at the hospital was so uninterested, but [also felt] that he had all the knowledge at his fingertips, he should have told us of [who was available] such as the occupational therapist, the speech therapist, the physiotherapist, and so on.

Julian echoes the apparently fortuitous process through which external help materialises, although he and his wife discovered an unexpected source of professional support:

Fortunately, [after I knew my diagnosis] I found that a colleague had knowledge of this disease and told me of the MNDA. My wife wrote to get details. In the meantime a neighbour of my mother's told her health visitor that she had a friend who might need help. The health visitor has been marvellous – someone you could actually talk to about housing, speech therapy, home helps etc. What concerns me most about all this is that the only practical advice and help we have received has come about by accident.

However great the professional intervention, and whatever the sources and effects of external information, one of the most striking aspects of direct familial involvement with MND/ALS is the extent to which there is an enormous reservoir of skill and developing expertise amongst those with MND/ALS, and their relatives. Thus Parks' comments above about the problems arising in the care of the person with MND/ALS through relatives and friends not being 'licensed and skilled' probably appears ironic to those engaged in such tasks. In this respect, expertise in the care of someone with MND/ALS, as well as those with other conditions, perhaps by definition is considered by professional health care staff to be something that is only possessed through organised study, success in which is demonstrated by objective and collectively validated assessments. Indeed, expertise is precisely not something it is thought can be gained solely by everyday experience, however telling the situation – although expertise might be enhanced by such experience. There is also another problem in relation to considering the skills developed by people with MND/ALS and their relatives as 'expertise', and that is because not only are their skills experientially rather than professionally developed, but usually, apart from exceptional situations, skills are focused on one individual rather than a group of those in similar situations. Thus, in the former situation, it might be (professionally) argued that the generalisability to others of the knowledge that might be gained was limited.

The implications of these arguments here is that the bulk of the burden of daily management of people with MND/ALS is almost always in their own hands or, as we shall argue, those of family and/or friends even in the later more demanding stages of the condition. Professional interventions of whatever kind are likely to be (in people's own terms) sporadic, and usually limited in time and effect. In this sense, 'the ongoing partnership' by professional health care staff with people with MND/ALS and their relatives mentioned above, is not just one between the expertise of the professional and the personal objectives of the family concerned with MND/ALS, but a partnership based on mutual skills – one gained by professional qualifications and the other by hard-won experience.

CREATING AND MAINTAINING ORDER IN THE EARLY STAGES OF MND/ALS

Managing MND/ALS can be considered to be attempting to create and maintain order – in the body and in the home – in the face of formidable pressures and processes tending continually to undermine and demolish that order. As most people with MND/ALS, and their relatives, manage their condition at home, at least initially, the problem is how to integrate a viable home life with the considerable potential for disorder. The extent of alterations that are made to fixed equipment, to clothes, to ordinary domestic routines, to the use of space, and to social relationships as part of this process can be formidable. In a succinct way, Rachel lists just some of the relatively modest range of things – compared to other households – which she has done for her mother who was recently diagnosed with MND/ALS:

> We had a couple of grab handles installed; a telephone she could take around the house; bought her easy-on easy-off clothing; an electric foot muff; firm shoes with flat soles; a walking frame with wheels (she found that a great help and very safe); a stool to sit on in the shower; higher 3 pin plugs with handles on; special scissors and several kitchen aids available from the local authority.

A more formidable list of changes, but over a far longer period, also indicates the degree of adaptation which may be required – although Joel was fortunate to have a job, and an employer, who enabled him to continue to work for many months after his diagnosis and when his symptoms were restricting many of his activities:

Year 1	Had just moved to new house; first signs of weakness in right arm in January; cellulitis in right leg February; consulted doctor re weakness late August; diagnosis late September, now affecting both arms.
Year 2	New house suitable for disabled people; downstairs bedroom/bathroom with plenty of room for equipment; near shops, work, school; first sign of weakness in legs in July; ceased driving; From March I was unable to dress or feed myself.
Year 3	January commenced half time working; February started falling over; started using wheelchair; unable to wash or shave self; social services supplied system to enable me to control the lights, telephone, television, radio, front door lock and intercom; MNDA supplied page turner; computer/communications software from speech therapist after a visit to a communication aids centre; social services also supplied electric rising and reclining easy chair.
Year 4	January, ceased working somewhat reluctantly, but had been ineffective for some time. February ceased walking, swallowing difficulties started. Unable to do anything for self except with control system, page turner, electric wheelchair, computer/communications software, which require setting up, adjustment and fitting by an attendant.
Year 5	Further swallowing difficulties, frequent choking and coughing, some breathing problems, voice weak, uncomfortable sitting, reclining, lying down. Control system attached to electric wheelchair using tray fixing point. New computer/communications software financed by MNDA.

Although it may appear an obvious point, all of the things mentioned by Rachel and Joel require changes in previous routines. Each one has been arrived at, not only through the perceived inadequacy of those routines, but through a process of advice seeking, experimentation and trial and error. Thus, in many cases, a solution to a problem does not just appear, it has to be worked at, developed and fine tuned. Even those things which may be recommended by 'expert others', and particularly any professional staff involved, also almost certainly have to be modified albeit in some minor way to adapt to the situation. As we noted above, whereas the experience of people with MND/ALS and their relatives is not often regarded by professional staff as transferable or generalisable, the problem with the generalised expertise of those staff may itself be considered by people with the disease not to be easily applicable to the very particular circumstances in which they find themselves. In other words, professional staff may find it difficult to understand and to work within the particular familial sense of order and priorities to which they are applying that expertise.

One of the most obvious areas in which major differences occur between community-based therapists and people with MND/ALS and their families is in relation to physiotherapy. For many people with MND/ALS, regular and continuing physiotherapy is considered to be essential to their well-being through the regular maintenance of their declining muscle capacity and strength. On the contrary, it appears that physiotherapists in general, within their professional framework and judgement, have a more focused and limited view of their role. In the case of Josie, this has been a very particular problem for her husband that has required home-made solutions:

> I wished someone had helped me when his physiotherapy was stopped, this is one thing that must be carried on with when possible. We had to work out our own way of getting the necessary exercise. We have two ropes with loops on hanging from the ceiling, we put his hands in each day and work his arms up and down. We also have a rubber grip on the grab rail where we can get his arms moving the other way in and out.

Josie's case, together with that of Edward mentioned earlier in this chapter, suggests that the way that this kind of professional care is organised does not fit in easily with the kind of domestic order which people with MND/ALS and their families are trying, in many cases desperately, to establish. The organisation of the home as a place in which sickness is managed is a very complicated affair. For it is not just creating the easiest environment in which technical solutions to major symptomatic problems can be accomplished, it is trying to maintain at the same time a viable 'home' in which – in most cases – others, as well as the person with MND/ALS, can continue to have a special relationship with each other and to a place, which is not possible elsewhere. As many of these latter aspects of 'home' are likely to be individual, idiosyncratic and precisely not amenable to professional assessment, let alone professional support, there are always likely to be tensions in the process of jointly managing health care for the person with MND/ALS.

FROM MANAGING THE PRESENT TO REFLECTING ON THE PAST AND TO THE FUTURE

As we noted at the beginning of this chapter the paradox of managing the detail of the present is that it invariably also focuses attention on the future. Moreover, such attention is not just on future symptoms and their management, but on their impact on all aspects of life and, conversely, of all aspects of life on them. Penny's description of the effects of one of her current symptoms of MND/ALS immediately triggers even more painful concerns about all aspects of her life:

> Each time I fall, I seem to know that I am about to go over and I am unable to 'break' the fall and lessen the blow. I don't know why this is, some people may not be able to understand, but this is how it has happened with me. For others it might have been 'old age' coming on. I have myself gone through the 'change of life' and this could have been what the next stage of life was! But it is only the 'next stage' for MND/ALS sufferers I have now found out, or at least for me as a sufferer.

> I have had a lot of help from doctors, a health visitor, social worker, and an occupational therapist –and eventually a physiotherapist when required. [However] friends and relatives have gradually tapered off – as if they were all waiting around to see what would happen – then realising they may feel obliged to 'do' something so have receded into the background again. Not least my husband – he cannot love me nor understand the meaning of the word – or he would not be so unkind to me ... [S]o began the decline in our relationship, so much so, that I am unable to trust his motives and am separating from him, so that he may be relieved of me as a burden to him and that he may become a better friend than a lover.

The issue of what the disease means in the context of close relationships is an ever present one, not least because, although Penny found it difficult to obtain the support she wished from anyone, actual or potential sources of support are something of a preoccupation.

For Penny, MND/ALS has clearly been a problem too far in her relationship with her husband, and even despite her worrying symptoms she is taking what some others might feel is a relatively drastic step to reorientate her life, and to re-establish control over it as far as possible. Others who are living on their own with MND/ALS are not so sure that the hopes of Penny will be borne out. After giving a lengthy list of an increasing range of equipment and services that she has required over a fifteen-month period with the disease, Ann gives a rather morose assessment of her future:

Month 1	Joined M.N.D. Association.
Month 2	I moved to a ground floor flat, that would take a wheelchair, because steps and stairs had become very difficult.
Month 3	Started at a Day Centre 1 day a week to try computers.
Month 10	Stayed in Assessment Centre to see what additional help needed.
Month 11	I have bought a small electrical stimulation machine and the nurses are starting to come in every day to get the electrodes either side of my spine to try & relieve some of the pain in my back & legs. Special mattress supplied by the M.N.D.A.
Month 12	Reclining armchair.
Month 13	Electric Wheelchair.
Month 15	(Hopefully) shower unit to be installed.

Overall living on my own I fear what is in front of me. I find that people who would visit me and so on, don't now that they know that I have M.N.D. I feel very alone at times.

However, for those who have partners, a common response as MND/ALS intervenes, whatever the day-to-day tensions involved and whatever the strains and stresses, is that of a very matter-of-fact relationship between long-standing partners – at least from the side of the person with MND/ALS – which is made easier if the course of the disease, as in Walter's case, is relatively slow:

At the moment I have wasted muscles in the hands, but I have still got a fairly good grip in both. But both thighs have wasted along with the buttocks. I am in continuous pain either sitting or walking, which is difficult for me. However I have a part time job driving. I have had to get a full medical report from my doctor to show that I can still use my mobility in legs & arms. [However] my mental attitude is good, I don't spend my time moping or worrying about what might happen in the future. My driving job might help in this as I travel all over the country, if I was sat at home all day it might be different . . . From what I've seen, everyone is slightly different. There are different varieties or strains of it. Mine appears to be progressing at a lot slower rate than many other peoples. My wife is fully aware of what problems could lie ahead, but says we'll deal with them as they arise –my thinking too!

Apart from some current problematic symptoms, Walter seems to have what one might describe as a modestly optimistic view of the future, although it might be more appropriate to consider that he is just living life as it comes, which Ted is doing but with a meticulous approach to all aspects of his situation:

It is difficult to think too much about the future but rather take every day as it comes and concentrate on the positive aspects, things could be worse. As a result of my job I always analyze and plan everything and so it is at home too. I keep a medical diary of progress. I make and re-make endless lists of things to do or actions which must be done or things I would like to do. I have many varied interests and am trying to find interests that I can do on my own.

For younger men with MND/ALS, in particular, financial worries about mortgages combined with those about their families are a special burden, as Daniel relates:

I have a mortgage of £29,000 and a loan of £6,000 (5 years to go) to pay off. This seems to be our greatest concern as staying in our house seems vital – i.e. we love it here, we like the neighbourhood, close to school, work, shops, bus, apart from which we have spent over £30,000 doing it up and it's now finished and perfect for us.

Such concerns may also centre on the more intimate parts of their relationship with their partners:

Sex between us has been a problem since the diagnosis . . . I think I can still function in this area of life but not to a level that would give any brownie points. We have been faithful partners and it has always disappointed me my wife has missed so much in this intimate area. I do not know if there is anything I can do in practical terms. I have not given up hope and intend working on the situation, where possible.

In many respects, the range and nature of most of these concerns are strikingly ordinary. Most people have concerns about some aspects of their future, they have concerns about their relationships, about their work, about themselves and about their children. It is the fact that living with MND/ALS appears to heighten and illuminate these concerns with a spotlight, and, just as significantly, propels people to think them through in an accelerated and more decisive way. The anxiety is it may not be possible to defer decisions any longer about those issues which, for a range of reasons, have been left on one side as other components of life proceeded. Life has become finite, and a controllable quality of life even more so, thus action now becomes more pressing. The extent to which positive contact can be maintained with people outside the home is important in this process.

LIVING WITH MND/ALS IN A PUBLIC WORLD

Despite recent major publicity about MND/ALS, and what might be construed as a high public profile for the problems of people with the disease, many of the accounts in this analysis document the difficulties experienced by people with MND/ALS in public settings – particularly in relation to how particular symptoms are socially 'read' and responses are made to them. To a large extent this is not surprising for, as we have already argued, symptoms or diseases do not have a socially detached or objective existence; they are locked into a set of assumptions about who people are, and about what being normal or abnormal is. Even if more 'objective' information is provided in the public domain about the medical and other aspects of MND/ALS, there is no guarantee that such information will affect public responses to people with the condition in the way intended or argued for. Primarily, reactions to those with MND/ALS in the public domain are conditioned initially by what are generally deemed to be normal expectations of people of a particular age, gender and disposition. In this respect, even the reaction of people who were previously relatively close, people at work or friends, can be disappointing, as they find it difficult to manage the intrusion of MND/ALS in their friendship. Wendy says:

[her husband's] work friends did not call because he could not speak. He had his note pad by his side, what were they afraid of? Perhaps they could not cope with illness. How very sad!

Sometimes, even when friends did call, it was obviously a problem how to manage the situation, as Irene recounts:

Friends would ask 'Are you feeling better?' when she was obviously deteriorating daily. She much preferred the sort of visitor who would keep her up to date with current happenings and did not expect her to do much talking which she found exhausting. Almost everyone took her chocolates which she couldn't eat, even though she frequently mentioned that she couldn't eat sweet things because she choked on them.

Joan has some good advice in this situation, but it seems to conflict a little with the point that has just been made:

When my husband was diagnosed . . . it didn't take very long to find out who my real friends were. The majority of 'my friends' ignored me or said things like 'I have wanted to call but I didn't know what to say.' It is really very simple, 'Hello, how are you,' if you really care, the rest just comes naturally . . . I have one real friend, she calls and asks about me first. She knows that I am the same person, just circumstances have made major changes. She insists I get out at least once a week for lunch. She just drops by to give me a hug. She will bring dinner by once in a while to give me a break from cooking. She also gives little gifts for no reason. She lets me know that I'm important in her life and she's always there for me, no matter what. Don't worry that what you say may seem inadequate, what's important is that you're there and the person whose caring doesn't feel abandoned just because others make her feel that way.

In the wider public world certain kinds of symptoms may indeed be seen as odd, strange or bizarre, especially those which can occur in MND/ALS, which are described medically as signs of 'emotional lability'. In Jock's situation he found this particularly difficult:

I'd like to mention . . . bulbar related symptoms, namely exaggerated laughing, crying, exaggerated anger and surprise. They seem to take me by surprise when they occur and laughing in particular can be very embarrassing when it becomes uncontrollable. It's quite hilarious with family and friends but not so in public!

I'm starting to feel like a maniac when travelling by public transport and suddenly bursting into prolonged peels of laughter.

At a more general level, Helen had problems because she 'looked well' in the early stages of MND/ALS :

I have dealt with problems [with others] by honesty, going to the source by head of department or company, explaining even though I look well I really am ill, and even though I am trying to continue a 'normal' life as much as possible and in doing so help to keep me more normal. However then odd things happen to remind me that I do have MND/ALS – a leg cramp, crying or laughing when I should not. Getting angry, and after, depressed, when people don't understand me. I try to, and am able to make myself heard, but some people are so patronising, some shout, some think I am crazy. It is tiring at first, battling with other people, but 'stick to your guns', and keep on explaining and so on, and ignore people who talk 'over you'.

Social scientists, following Goffman (1964), have widely reported the public problems that people with many medical conditions have, and have often used the idea of 'stigma' either to denote social disapproval of particular diseases or of particular symptoms, such that people may be driven into private rather than public lives by such disapproval. One of the latest analyses using the idea of stigma is that of Nijhof (1995) who focuses his attention on the problems arising in public settings for people with another serious neurological condition – Parkinson's disease. He argues that many people with this disease, by virtue of their resulting physical mannerisms and difficulties in speech, break normal social expectations, and thus are seen as 'deviant' and socially 'shamed' by others. Therefore:

as a consequence of this shame, the informants speak of a split of their life world, and their inclination towards retreat from the public into the private. Parkinson's disease in this pattern of interpretation is the illness of shameful withdrawal from public life.

(1995: 202)

Such an analysis could be just as applicable to people with MND/ALS – as the case of Tony, relayed by his wife, suggests:

We stopped going out for a drink because with Tony's difficulty in walking and slurred speech people thought he was drunk. One night we went out Tony fell and cut his nose. We had only been in the club about half an hour everyone just looked at him laid out on the floor. I had to explain about MND/ALS. Tony said he could not face the embarrassment. We did go out for a drink a few times when he was in his wheelchair, but Tony could not lift the glass to his mouth so my friends husband gave him his drink. It became obvious that Tony was uncomfortable with this so we decided to stay in from then on.

Often the ways in which difficult situations with others are managed is with dry and ironic humour. Tony's wife, following her experiences above, indicates the strategy:

I made a point of putting him through as little embarrassment as I could by making a joke about everything. We shared a lot of laughter through his illness, even when he became totally dependent on me. I once threw his dinner against a wall because he wouldn't open his mouth for me to feed him, he sat there laughing whilst I cleaned the mess up. Every time we had visitors after that he wanted me to tell them about it, it became funnier the more times I told it.

It takes a robust and direct approach to ordinary social encounters to be able to deal with the situations that Wendy describes so amusingly:

there was 'The Wheelchair'. We would go out shopping with it in the boot. But I wasn't very good at getting it unfolded. That was when I learnt to smile at strong young men. The one in Coventry was stunning but turned out to be a non-English-speaking Spaniard. The ensuing conversation was like an episode from 'Fawlty Towers!' The same day there was suddenly a man-hole cordoned off right across the pavement. Four lusty Americans hoisted Derek and chair high above their heads and cheered as they lowered him on the other side. He nervously smiled his thanks. Then there was the incident in the supermarket (before they had these trolleys which clip on to wheelchairs) I'd left him where he could see down the aisles while I shopped. When I returned, he was quietly chuckling to himself. 'What's the joke?' 'D'you see that old girl just going out? She said to me "Are you alright, luv? You look just like me poor 'ubby did just before he was took!"' And in another supermarket, when we got jammed at the cash-out, they said 'Come on, girls!' and bodily lifted all the fittings off the floor. 'Any time, dear.' 'Aren't people kind?' I said. 'That's because they are bloody glad it's not them' Derek said.

These quotations demonstrate that the management of MND/ALS involves both negotiating the catalogue of technical difficulties that arise in everyday life as the condition progresses, but – just as important – negotiating the challenge of social and personal relationships in which those difficulties are defined and placed. At each stage, people with the disease and their family members have to work through these issues with each other, as well as with what may become an increasing army of others concerned with health care who pay more or less helpful, and more or less sporadic, visits offering what they hope is useful and reassuring support. In the end, however, the integration of all these processes into life with MND/ALS is undertaken by the person with MND/ALS, and those informally caring for and supporting them.

Chapter 5

The desperate search for causes and cures for motor neurone disease

SEARCHING FOR THE CAUSE

Although biomedically the causes of most types of MND/ALS are only beginning to be unravelled, with a likely genetic susceptibility compounded by environmental factors of some kind being a significant component, the quest for explanations in their personal histories by people with MND/ALS and their families as to why they have individually fallen prey to this condition is intense. Such a quest is a normal process that operates in relation to any untoward event, especially illness, which disrupts the usual flow of people's lives. In societies in Europe and North America in particular, where the focus is on the relatively autonomous role and personal standing of individuals, attention is especially drawn to those elements for which those individuals might have some (moral) responsibility. In this process the focus is not only on explanation, but, as Harris points out, also on interpretation:

> whatever the institutional contextualisation [hospitals, clinics, etc.], illness and injury must remain events in personal histories. As such they call everywhere not only for explanation but also for interpretation . . . Both explanation [identifying a cause for an event] and interpretation [identifying a reason for it] imbue an event with meaning. They differ importantly however. Explanation deals with elements and processes locally taught as truths about the way the world works. Interpretation suffuses events with evaluative significance. Explanation is about mechanism while interpretation is about morality, broadly conceived.
>
> (1989: 4)

To identify a probable cause (in Harris's terms an explanation) is

one thing, to identify why this happened (in Harris's terms an interpretation) is another. Interpretations in this sense are critical
because they place the cause in social and personal context – why
such a juxtaposition of events occurred and one's responsibility for
that juxtaposition.

For most people with MND/ALS, with long lives there is much
to interrogate in order to reveal the patterns which are perceived as
leading to the disease. The reservoir of possible factors is huge, and
their potential relationships to each other even more complex. For
some people, the 'narrative reconstruction' (Williams 1984) which
they undertake of those aspects of their lives that they feel have led
to their present predicament with MND/ALS is a relatively open
process. There is no neat and obvious pathway that can be
recounted from a single defined event to the MND/ALS, or even
from a trajectory which links several possible aetiological events. In
such cases, the MND/ALS remains a puzzle with few obvious clues
that might be targeted, partly because early events or circumstances
may be seen as so distant from the first symptoms of the disease –
often by a matter of decades – that their aetiological significance is
for most people questionable. In addition, in terms of possible
causative factors, people with MND/ALS may feel these early
events or circumstances to be counterbalanced by other lifestyle
factors, a countervailing view of causation in which subsequent
positive lifestyles may have cancelled out other earlier negative
influences on health and illness. In these cases, the account
produced by the person with MND/ALS is essentially one which is
offered for external corroboration and interpretation, as in Fred's
rather terse narrative of his life before MND/ALS:

> Born in 3rd October 1919; father 29 and mother 28; in my pre-
> teenage years I got untreated 'ague' from a foreign mosquito;
> started work at 14; severe sinusitis from age 20 to 35; had boils in
> various locations during the war; accident to back in 1951; acci-
> dent to left arm which broke three bones in 1953; illness in Spain
> in 1975 due to untreated sewage in sea; retired 1984; chiropractor
> worked on my back; prostrate operation May 1987; consulted the
> neurologist and diagnosed in December 1990; lifelong non-
> smoker; not alcoholic; not obese (80kgs); no drug abuse; not
> homosexual; no varicose veins; hobbies and interests – motor
> cycling from 1935 to 1964; ice skating club member; occupation
> skilled wood turner.

Reading into Fred's narrative, he clearly feels that although a number of problematic events – accidents and illnesses – have occurred throughout his life, his moral standing in his approach to his life is such that it almost seems unjust, as well as relatively inexplicable, that he has subsequently been diagnosed with MND/ALS. To put it another way, there seems to be no real reason, in his terms, for his MND/ALS. According to the moral code of many older people who have lived what they have considered to be upright lives, often in the face of considerable hardship or other difficulty, they feel strongly that they do not deserve the additional burden of MND/ALS. Moreover, this MND/ALS occurs, as we have noted previously, at a time when the rigours of a working life should be almost behind them. However, although they may feel this way, such people are not used to life being 'fair' or 'just', thus MND/ALS becomes one more cross to bear. Percy expresses the point succinctly:

It is one of life's ironies that, having led a blameless life with no smoking, drinking, drugs or other debaucheries, one ends up with a perfectly healthy body but is otherwise a zombie.

For relatives in particular, trying to make sense of how and why a husband or wife, or father or mother, has become affected by the disease, the puzzle may be even greater as they try to piece together long lives of which they may only have known a part. Tom's wife is trying as best she can to examine his life and reach for factors she feels might be implicated in the MND/ALS, but it is a bit of a struggle. The most promising lines of enquiry for her seem to be in relation to Tom's family:

None of us thought he had ever had any serious illness. His weakness in his legs we put down to a cartilage operation, that in his hands as the effects of accidents. Tom lived a very cheerful, happy life, even during his illness. Had been a member of the local Operatic Society and excellent at singing, dancing and acting. He had never been known to take any medication. He was very fond of Polo mints. I recently noticed a wedding photograph (1966) in which his left index finger was only bent at top joint. His height was 5′7″, and his weight 10–10½ stone. In 1976 I noticed Jack stooped, his mother stated that his father had similar condition. Father died 10th April 1962, 66 yrs old – death certificate – Heart failure due to pneumoconiosis and emphysema. Mother died 12th October 1979, 81 yrs old – death certificate – Heart failure. There was a history of asthma in Tom's mother and sister.

The view in such accounts that there may be, or indeed perhaps is, a family connection through a family 'weakness' or 'constitutional' problem is an interesting commentary on how people may, in their interpretation, draw on what they perceive to be the interlocking symptoms or illnesses of family members. Given the latest research on the aetiology of MND/ALS which increasingly implicates genetic factors in the condition, the coincidence of this traditional 'lay' view of one of the origins of family illnesses with recent biomedical findings is quite striking. In addition, in these accounts there is, to some degree, an attempt to evaluate a life in terms of its moral and life style qualities, and to reach into them to draw some broad conclusions about their relationship to MND/ALS.

For others the origins of MND/ALS are located in much more specific factors, whose traumatic nature seems to link naturally into the chronologically later trauma of the disease, and indeed there is still some doubt (and hope) about the status of the diagnosis of MND/ALS:

I was working on a water pipe that . . . unknown to me had an electrical short, when both of my hands made contact with the water pipe I was unable to let go because of the electrical current flowing through the pipe. After what I estimate to be 7 to 10 seconds I was able to break loose and fell to the floor. Although dizzy and shaken I never lost consciousness and had no visible burns. After taking a few hours off I went back to work feeling very lucky to apparently be O.K. I had some arm pain for a couple of days but that went away. About a month later I noticed my right index finger and thumb were weak I told my employer about this and he sent me to a physiotherapist thinking I may have hurt something when I fell to the floor. The physiotherapist treated me for a couple of months to no avail. In fact now I was having spasms in my right hand and my leg muscles felt tight. By December my right hand was so bad I lost my job . . . Some time later I was sent to see a neurologist . . . who indicated that my symptoms were consistent with what you would see with MND/ALS. [This] neurologist told me I was a textbook case of hand to hand electrocution . . . and that it will look just like

MND/ALS but hopefully it would . . . level off. Unfortunately it never did level off and the symptoms have progressed . . . Fast forwarding to the present I walk with the help of a walker, I have major atrophy and severe weakness in my upper body, atrophy in my hips, leg weakness, fasciculations, speech difficulty, minor swallowing and saliva problems, all, of course, classic MND/ALS symptoms.

Trauma of one kind or another has featured regularly in epidemiological studies of people's perceptions of the origins of their MND/ALS. Such trauma, in terms of accidents, broken bones, electric shocks, are significant life events and are particularly likely both to be remembered and to be linked to other later life events, whether they are of illness or of other kinds. In a case such as this, both the nature of the episode itself and the proximity of the 'MND/ALS-like' symptoms draw the two inexorably together. Indeed, it is possible that the two interpretations of the same event are correct. The condition may be both a case of delayed neurological effects from an electric shock, and also a case of classic MND/ALS triggered by this trauma. However, biomedical classification systems do not easily operate with such multiple interpretations for, as Christakis (1997) argues, all the emphasis is on separating out and clearly distinguishing individual conditions in their 'pure' or 'typical' form.

None the less, whilst traumas or difficulties in proximity to the onset of MND/ALS may be an important additional associative factor, they do not always need to be perceived to be close to the development of symptoms in order to be considered to have an aetiological effect. Given current environmental concerns, as well as public discussions of the pernicious effects of a wide range of toxic substances on health and more focused discussions on possible links between MND/ALS and such substances, most people's lives provide a rich source of occasions or circumstances when contact has been made with potential health hazards. Both 'natural' and 'unnatural' substances or situations may be deemed to be candidates. In particular, too much contact with nature, such as with farm animals and in farming settings, or too little contact – through living in towns, working in factories and using dangerous chemicals. Sometimes the two perceptions combine – as in contacts with chemicals used in farming settings. Dan is seeking to explain the source of his wife's MND/ALS and has produced, in effect, a list of many natural as well as other possibilities:

> Most of her life was spent on a farm . . . Throughout her life she helped on the farm, spending a lot of time milking the cows as well as dealing with the poultry. She has been in close contact almost all her life with animals and it has been usual to have at least one dog and cat in the home . . . Until the late 1950s she drank untreated milk from the farm cows . . . Near the farm were paint and metal-hardening factories. Some chemicals were also produced there and chemicals were used to spray the crops. She lived on a farm which also grew fruit and sprays were used on the trees. For most of her life the water used was from a deep bore and not from the mains. There was an extensive outbreak of polio in her area . . . in the late 1940s and cases were diagnosed two/three miles from the home. A lot of her life was spent in old farmhouses and these . . . were damp, cold and draughty. Heating was by wood fire mainly and there was an Aga burning anthracite and before that a paraffin cooking stove. Paraffin lamps were used. The piping was galvanised.

In the search for explanations, there is the hope, only very occasionally realised, that a little known but curable infectious disease might be responsible for the MND/ALS signs and symptoms. Charlotte is hoping that this may be the case with her husband's condition:

> Because of the rather unusual nature of my husband's symptoms and progression, and because he has travelled so extensively, often in very rough conditions, in almost all Third World countries . . . his neurologist [has] suggested that he consult an expert in tropical medicine to see if by any chance he might have some very rare tropical disease rather than MND/ALS (or in addition to MND/ALS). This suggestion is prompted by the fact that about 3 months after noticing neurological symptoms (foot drop, ataxia) he also had a bout of hepatitis that could not be identified. That has more or less resolved, but the thinking is that he may have picked up some weird virus, perhaps in Africa, that has led to an autoimmune response causing the motor neurone problems. Since he also has some sensory . . . problems in the feet and legs, as well as terrible pain in the legs that is not controlled with [name of drugs], it is thought that there might possibly be something else going on.

The issue of exhaustively exploring the lexicon of diseases for the possible intervention of a rare condition which might mimic the signs and symptoms of MND/ALS is one which evokes strong medical responses one way or another. In the same recently edited text, one neurologist feels that a major problem in many neurologists' clinical approach to MND/ALS is their tendency to perform legions of exclusionary tests which are not justifiable on the basis of the clear clinical symptoms presented (Bradley 1994: 23), whilst Norris argues for an extensive investigation – even if the clinical signs are relatively clear – and argues that:

> Even after an exhaustive apparently negative . . . [series of investigations], the attending physician should always maintain the possibility, however slight, of some other diagnosis.
>
> (ibid.: 32)

For most people with a provisional or even a firm diagnosis of the disease, their preference would certainly be for a continuing sceptical and investigative approach to the person with MND/ALS, for – in their eyes – no other diagnosis could have such a profoundly unwelcome course and outcome.

Two other major approaches that people with MND/ALS may have to understanding the causes of their disease are rather different in character. One of these, and in many respects the most common, revolves around the idea of 'stress' in one form or another. 'Stress' has become a frequent way of explaining many forms of illness in modern society. There is a paradox about discussing stress however. On the one hand, the word and its generic implications form a common currency and an everyday discourse which 'everyone understands'; on the other hand, the reference points of stress – what causes it, and indeed its specific consequences – in terms of particular illnesses or diseases can be considered to be quite different. For some people with MND/ALS, there is no doubt that what they consider as stressors in their lives formed a significant component of the cause of their disease. For example, Christine not only links a particularly stressful job with one of her most distressing symptoms, but also feels that in general stress is the only reasonable explanation of her condition, for even her period abroad did not – she believes – expose her to untoward factors:

> Looking back with hindsight I have often wondered whether the loss of speech may not have been an unfortunate psychological

reaction to my feeling about my job situation over the last couple of years, coupled with the natural stresses of the work. This would not of course account for the other physical developments. Otherwise stress of one sort or another is the only factor I can regard as a possible contributor to the contraction of the disease as, in my recollection, I have never experienced or been exposed to anything other than normal childhood complaints or unusual diets, even in India in wartime where life was very civilised in my immediate surroundings.

For other people stress is not only a reasonable explanation, it appears that the MND/ALS or some other such condition is an inevitable result of an almost endless series of troubles and disasters. Carol writes about the lengthy set of difficulties which have plagued her life:

My father collapsed and died with a heart attack, [and my] husband and I stayed with my mother for 3 months to help her get over it . . . When I took a full time job after a few months I kept getting dizzy attacks and I had to leave because the Doctor wouldn't let me go back full time. Then three years later my husband went out for a walk and didn't come back, so I contacted the police and then late that night I was told that he had been admitted to a MENTAL HOSPITAL. I was devastated. I visited him nearly every day for many months, occasionally having him home for some week-ends. Life then was taken one day at a time . . . [After a short period at home] he was taken back into a mental hospital, and then he got Parkinson's Disease, and eventually . . . [his problems] went to his lungs, and died . . . All this time I had been under the doctor.' [Carole then recounts how her mother then died, she was made redundant from her part-time job, and lost a close friend through cancer. These problems were then followed with a complicated series of over 30 separate hospital investigations for a range of serious symptoms over a two-year period, with various diagnoses. Finally she received her diagnosis from a leading neurologist. As Carole puts it] 'Dr X told me that I had M.N.D. on top of my other troubles!'

It is hard not to feel sympathetic with the view that at least some of Carole's tribulations can be explained biomedically as well as subjectively with reference to the catalogue of events to which she has been subject. However, as stress has become such a ubiquitous idea through which many (perhaps most) personal troubles are perceived, Harris argues that we must be aware of the particular ways in which the idea is used as a way of understanding illness in modern society. It has become, as he puts it, a 'medico-moral' term in which various events and circumstances are perceived as acting on, what he describes as, the 'psychologised self' to produce illness (1989: 6–7). In this process, as Carole's account indicates, social relationships are particularly important and, when they are problematic, are considered particularly dangerous to future health.

Scientists and clinicians, reflecting on the wide range of ways in which people account for their MND/ALS, might be tempted to argue that the aetiological ideas represented in these accounts are not only substantially at variance with scientific ideas, but are of little value for formal research – whatever value they may have for people with the disease as a means of understanding their own situation. However, such a view underestimates the vast range of candidate causative factors in MND/ALS which scientists themselves have explored, and indeed are currently exploring, and overestimates the separation of scientific ideas from everyday ideas about the origins of MND/ALS. Apart from the central role of stress as a causative factor in illness through mind–body interaction – which itself is now being explored through the relatively new sub-discipline of psycho-neuro-immunology – many of the other ideas which are mentioned are close to those of current scientific interest. The role of family/constitutional factors echoes scientific concerns with genetic/inherited variables; the role of environmental hazards reflects that of scientific exploration of neurotoxins; and there is a long history of epidemiological and clinical concern with the relationship between trauma and the onset of MND/ALS.

THE SEARCH FOR A CURE

The role, power and expectations of modern scientific medicine are such that it is difficult for many people to countenance that any condition is incurable, particularly one which has a fatal outcome. Scientific medicine with its apparently inexorable and cumulative conquest of a wide range of hitherto intractable conditions, together with a repertoire of almost daily reports of advances and 'breakthroughs', suggests that every condition is within its sights and, imminently, within its grasp. Not to have the possibility of a cure for MND/ALS can therefore be literally unbelievable. In Chapter 3, we demonstrated how difficult it was for people with MND/ALS, as well as their relatives, to digest this information, not only because it precipitated a tragic human dilemma, but because it juxtaposed what had previously been considered to be the curative power of scientific medicine to its impotence in the case of this disease.

The requirements which are apparently imposed by scientific methods on people with MND/ALS, who might otherwise wish to seek alternative therapeutic options outside those of scientific medicine, are formidable. The randomised controlled trial (RCT) is the method of choice for scientifically evaluating potential therapies. Although there are various forms of trial designs, an RCT requires an intervention group (who will be given the potential therapy), and a control group (who will not receive the potential therapy, but will often receive an inactive substance – a placebo). Furthermore, people (patients) will be randomly allocated to either the intervention group or the control group without knowing to which group they have been allocated, and that knowledge will also not be available to the researchers carrying out the trial (the trial is thus conducted 'blind'). Only at a chosen point – possibly one, two, or more years from the beginning of the trial – will the trial be 'unblinded' to assess whether the potential therapy has performed better on the criteria selected than the placebo substance. Those criteria are often a matter of substantial debate but could, in relation to MND/ALS, be survival, or carefully measured functional changes, or 'quality of life' changes, or targeted physiological changes. Only if the potential therapy shows a statistically significant positive difference on one or more of these criteria (compared to the placebo) would it be deemed to be useful in treating MND/ALS. However, almost certainly further RCT's would be needed to test whether the positive results were 'real', or obtained through chance, or derived through some problem in the original trial design or operation. In addition, there would need to be studies of appropriate dose levels and modes of administration of the potential therapy. Even to reach the point of full evaluation through an RCT in this way may require several years of development in the laboratory, through tests on animals, and initial safety testing on humans.

For people with MND/ALS with a limited, broadly predictable, but exactly unknown lifespan ahead of them, these scientific requirements for testing new therapies are often problematic in major ways (Robinson 1990). First, the length of time taken, both to develop potential therapies and to evaluate them through an RCT, is likely to exceed many individual's lifespans. Second, the requirements for randomisation in many RCTs will mean that half of those participating in such trials will not receive the potential therapy at all, but due to 'blinding' processes will not know whether they have received the active agent or not. Third, the requirements for entry into such a trial – for example, in terms of age, disease state, and other simultaneously occurring conditions – may severely restrict who, out of all those with MND/ALS, can participate. Fourth, there may be other significant logistic issues for people with MND/ALS in terms of willingness to undergo major and continuing assessments, perhaps at distant institutions. Fifth, people who are participating may be required to forsake other possible therapeutic options for the duration of their involvement in the trial, and indeed be under substantial pressure to continue to participate until the end of the trial, even if they feel – or indeed are completely convinced – that they are not benefiting themselves from their role. And sixth, the obscure peer-reviewed processes (from a lay point of view) through which information about trial results may only gradually percolate to people with MND/ALS is slow and not readily accessible.

Despite such a substantial list of caveats which people with MND/ALS might have about involvement in clinical trials, the arguments of scientists and clinicians are that the RCT represents not just the best way of evaluating potential therapies in MND/ALS, it represents the only way of testing them. In this respect, there is both broad agreement amongst all mainstream scientists and clinicians that this is the way to proceed (Khabbaz and Roos 1994) and, at the same time, there is a very active attempt to dissuade people with MND/ALS from any other course of action. Although Glasberg has noted that:

> It will continue to be hard to discourage our patients from obtaining alternative treatments when we do not have any treatments available to either cure or significantly alter the course of the disease.

He still presses strongly for a range of procedures and supports to be put in place to persuade people with MND/ALS to participate in clinical trials, and indeed to discourage them from obtaining other (non-scientifically validated) treatment options (1994: 53–61).

There are many, particularly older people, with MND/ALS who would be grateful for the opportunity to participate in *any* clinical trial which might possibly give them the slightest hope of ameliorating their MND/ALS in even modest ways, almost whatever the 'terms and conditions' of participation. This is not so much a question of faith in science or medicine as, in their perception, the absence of any alternative possibility of redressing their disease. As Ivor writes:

> I am still walking around but my right foot has dropped; and my speech has totally gone, but my vocal chords seem O.K. . . . I will not give up, and [I will] try to live a normal life. Yes, I get scared when I think about this illness. Let's hope there will be a cure, not only for me, but for everyone. I would hope to be picked for any research or trials or tests – what have I got to lose!

For others, the scientific niceties of testing extensively and at length for the safety of potential therapies seems an inordinate luxury when the prospect of death, the ultimate unsafe experience, looms so large. For Kevin, his friend:

> who is on assisted breathing and is no longer able to swallow and [can] hardly talk, has strong feelings about the safety aspect . . . He feels that he isn't too concerned about . . . safety . . . since as in his case he doesn't have a future of health anyway . . . it will definitely go downhill. In fact, he would love to be the subject of non-scientific experimentation . . . he desperately wants more life, just for a while, to communicate specific things to his kids who are with his ex-wife, outside of easy visiting distance . . . How concerned are we about safety with this disease, and is it worth while [to experiment] just to learn something?

In the light of such arguments, the prospect of only receiving a placebo – a non-active therapy – in a clinical trial in the pursuance of the greater scientific good is not only disheartening, it seems to some with the disease an almost criminal act. A vigorous American account on an electronic bulletin board by someone with MND/ALS takes issue with the consistent use of placebos in North American trials on the disease:

> The FDA [the American Food and Drugs Administration]

authorizes drug trial protocols and will allow for parallel track, history controls, dose variances and placebo control studies. Of these forms of drug trials, the use of placebos borders on 'crimes against humanity'. In a disease such as MND/ALS, there has never been a therapy or cure/remission. For over 125 years, physicians have measured and observed the deaths of hundreds of thousands suffering from this horrific disease . . . the use of placebos in the terminally ill is the same as saying these people are 'expendable' . . . Claiming that placebos allow drug trials to proceed faster, cheaper and provide meaningful measurements ignores the humanity of those given 'false hope' by this research methodology.

Few individuals with MND/ALS would deliberately wish to accept a placebo, unless they have a considerable altruistic motivation which overrides other concerns. This balance between egoistic and altruistic concerns in placebo-controlled clinical trials is being more extensively discussed as recruitment for some such trials is becoming more difficult (Rosenberg 1993). However, the whole debate about the role of placebos could take a different direction if, as seems very possible, an active drug – already proven to have some effect on the course of MND/ALS – becomes the standard treatment in clinical trials in place of a placebo. Even so, the chance, however slim, of an additional positive effect may still be too tempting for some people with the disease to take such a standard treatment.

It is perhaps not surprising, through frustration with many elements of the clinical trials process, as well as dealing with the very pressing problem of keeping alive, that either instead of – or frequently in addition to – participation in such trials, people with MND/ALS engage in many (in conventional scientific terms) alternative therapeutic strategies. Involvement in such strategies may take many forms of which the general medical view is that they:

[unorthodox treatments], for MND/ALS have had a markedly negative effect on patients and families, who can deplete not only their financial resources but also their valuable time in undergoing these treatments. Even worse a feeling of hopelessness may set in to make patients avoid treatments at multidisciplinary clinics.

(Glasberg 1994: 61)

Such a view does not appear to take into account the complexity of decisions to engage in such actions and fails to note other forms of benefit which may be gained by people with MND and their relatives – and which operate outside the rationality of modern medicine (Good 1994). It also fails to appreciate the considerable intellectual, as well as emotional, energy which is often devoted to researching and developing reasons and rationales for particular interventions. These, and lay debates about them, often bear a close resemblance to conventional dense and detailed scientific arguments about particular approaches to the disease – indeed the protagonists would say they are one and the same. A notable case in point is the often impressive array of debates about the merits and deficiencies of retaining or removing amalgam dental fillings in relation to affecting the course of MND/ALS. For the most part, it is not the case, as some scientists appear to suppose, that people with MND/ALS unthinkingly and completely irrationally rush from one alternative strategy to another. Indeed, contrary to Glasberg's views above, the surprise may be that more people do not adopt alternative therapies which can be considerably *less* costly in many ways than all the various costs involved in still relatively ineffective scientific therapies.

CHANGING THE RESEARCH AGENDA: PEOPLE WITH MND/ALS AND THE ROLE OF THE WORLD WIDE WEB

Most people with MND/ALS, and most of the time until recently, were trebly disadvantaged in relation to expressing their detailed wishes about the research agenda in relation to the disease, let alone being able to exercise any significant control over it. First, as we have seen, the 'normal' authority of clinicians and scientists was such that their *bona fides* and their established approach to the aims as well as the management of research was relatively unquestioned. Second, most people with MND/ALS are older people whose generally deferential approach to established medical and other authority has further reinforced that authority. Third, and very particularly, the nature of the condition itself with its rapidly debilitating effects on mobility of any kind as well as on the usual means of interpersonal communication, has also often left any means of forcefully asserting their ideas and wishes about research to clinicians and scientists in jeopardy. However, the advent and recent use of the World Wide Web (the Internet), and especially electronic mailing lists, has begun to change the balance of power – and authority – between people with MND/ALS, scientists and clinicians, pharmaceutical companies developing potential therapies for MND/ALS, and other organisations which have traditionally had a relatively central and broadly unchallenged role in the care of people with MND/ALS – including patient organisations in the voluntary sector.

Given the communication difficulties which many people with MND/ALS face – which we shall explore in more detail in Chapter 6 – the use of various forms of computer-assisted communication is becoming increasingly widespread. Although such equipment is, for the most part, used in a local and particular context to assist communication between family members and others, in principle much is easily adaptable for broader communication to others outside the home. Indeed, three further factors – the increasingly restricted possibilities of social interaction outside the home, lengthy periods of time spent in one setting, and the adaptability of computer technology to control through even minute bodily movements (for example eye blinks) – make this possibility more likely.

Although the degree to which what might be described as extended computer technology is deployed by people with MND/ALS is still relatively limited in Britain, it has been estimated that approaching 25 per cent of all people with serious or terminal conditions in the United States now have direct or indirect access to World Wide Web resources. The importance of this development does not lie so much in the proportion of people with MND/ALS who have some immediate access to this resource, however, as it does in the ways in which the qualities and effects of use of the World Wide Web are changing the nature of the debate about the disease. In particular, it is changing ideas both about what 'information' about MND/ALS is: who can generate it; who can modify it, and above all who can control it. Conventionally, 'information' has been considered to be a neutral objective commodity in scientific medicine, and further has been something which has generally been seen to be generated and held by scientists and clinicians and released to patients and their families at appropriate times – decided largely by those scientists and clinicians.

Arksey's (1994) reflections on Fleck's (1935) analysis suggest that scientific knowledge is much more likely to have always been derived from a broader constituency of ideas and influences than scientists usually entertain, in which influences well beyond the academy, laboratory or clinic condition the nature of that knowledge. For Fleck, Arksey argues:

> medical facts are established by means of the exchange and circulation of ideas and practical experience between specialists, general practitioners and patients . . . [and] . . . a key implication of this perspective is that scientific knowledge is not 'discovered' by technical experts and then disseminated to a wider public, but that these audiences from the very beginning participate in verifying the knowledge in the first place.
>
> (1994: 448–9)

In this argument the role of lay people (for example, patients in medical settings) is important both, on the one hand, in raising issues which are subsequently pursued and often then appropriated by 'experts', and, on the other hand, lay people use and thereby validate experts and their knowledge. To put the point another way, there is a mutually significant process at work with lay people helping to construct the nature of expert knowledge, and experts trying to configure users, so that the former's knowledge is considered valid and relevant. Whilst Arksey and Fleck, and subsequently many sociologists of science, consider this process to have been operating continually, the newer electronic media provide an even more open and explicit avenue through which the mutual relationship between medical experts and lay people (patients) is made visible.

For those people with MND/ALS who have access to the World Wide Web, an extraordinarily rich tapestry of expert knowledge is (relatively) easily available, which may not only be accessed in general terms but can often be actively interrogated. Moreover, the usual personal and structural intermediaries to such knowledge – conventional libraries and librarians, the experts themselves (in the form of doctors and scientists), managerial structures (in the form of health service providers), and even voluntary organisations concerned with MND/ALS – are less able to control the process of acquisition of knowledge itself, even if they originally compiled the resource of information. Furthermore, other mechanisms in the form of electronic mailing lists now allow a relatively free exchange of views about all aspects of this knowledge largely unencumbered by the ministrations of conventional authority.

Two electronic mailing lists in particular have been very influential in constructing a different public set of agendas about the disease. The first is the ALSIG (Amyotrophic Lateral Sclerosis Interest Group) newsletter which has been compiled in digest form weekly for the past five years by Bob Broedel of the University of Florida, and has become available internationally both in current and archive form through the Centre for the Study of Health at Brunel University, London, as well as more recently through other North American sources. The second is an ALS Bulletin Board organised through the electronic service provider Prodigy in the United States. This Bulletin Board is not initially compiled in digest form before transmission, as is the ALSIG newsletter, but is a forum for instant electronic communication between individuals.

An analysis of the kinds of material discussed, distributed and debated on these mailing lists indicates that they are used for checking on their diagnostic status by people with MND; for the exchange of ideas and concerns over detailed issues of the management of MND/ALS at all stages of the disease; for reporting on individual histories of themselves or their relatives with the disease; for ascertaining from others their views on current or proposed therapies; for reporting on political, as well as scientific and medical, developments in MND/ALS; for challenging, and for lobbying for changes in the policies and practices of government, as well as medical, commercial and voluntary organisations; for giving information about the availability and progress of clinical trials and for, on occasions, coordinating preliminary findings through the reports of individuals on their experiences in trials; for discussing the organisation of clinical trials, and criteria for their evaluation and assessment; from time to time, for organising, through their contributors what scientists might describe as informal trials of potential therapies; for debates over the status of various conventional and unconventional ideas on the aetiology of MND/ALS, and for a wide range of other purposes.

The importance of this rapidly expanding interactive set of resources lies in its broadly democratic and egalitarian structure, in the sense that the information flow is relatively uncontrolled and contributions are relatively uncensored. Given the usual hierarchical structures within scientific medicine, through which attempts are often made to manage both the nature and extent of information, the use of the World Wide Web is relatively open, indeed, from the point of view of medical and other authority, its use is almost anarchic. It has become therefore very difficult for traditional health agencies and professionals to isolate a body of information as expert knowledge and to control its use. This situation, as Arksey indicates, represents a substantial threat to conventional expertise. Her analysis suggests the apparently expanding role of lay knowledge about MND/ALS through the World Wide Web and other sources, and the associated power gained from that knowledge, may be short-lived, even though initially:

> there is an opening for persons considered normally technically incompetent to acquire (lay) medical power with regard to the construction of scientific facts. At the same time, though, it might be the case that as specialists learn to recognise conditions originally identified by lay 'experts', they also appropriate them. As a consequence, experts are in a position to gain power over that domain and in the process delete the original authorship of the lay public from the acknowledged history. This point accords with medicine's disinclination to act in ways likely to threaten the authority and status of its power base.
>
> (1994: 464)

There have not only been serious concerns expressed by doctors and scientists about the role of the World Wide Web, and particularly electronic mailing lists in relation to MND/ALS, but explicit attempts to control and manage them. In relation to other conditions, this has occasionally occurred by sponsoring organisations reconstructing mailing lists or World Wide Web sites as solely or mainly for use by qualified professions, with prior censorship of material. However, the multiplicity of routes in and through these electronic media make such control difficult. Furthermore, in the case of MND/ALS, the use of these electronic media is likely to be persistent, growing and continuous, for they represent one of the very few ways in which those with advanced MND/ALS can communicate with some ease with others outside, for whom the momentum triggered by a dying trajectory to find the cause(s) and a cure is a major preoccupation. It is indeed to a discussion of the later stages of MND/ALS to which we now turn.

Chapter 6

Living and dying with motor neurone disease

TECHNIQUES, TECHNOLOGIES AND THE MANAGEMENT OF LIFE THREATENING SYMPTOMS

There is yet another paradox in relation to this disease which is full of paradoxes. For most people with the condition, as the seemingly inexorable progression continues, and points are reached sometimes sooner and sometimes later when symptoms threaten life, the more those symptoms require technical skills and expertise to manage them, the more they raise completely non-technical issues. Those issues are to do with the person at the heart of the disease, and the nature of their relationship to others, as well as to life itself. None the less, the technical management of MND/ALS generates a high level of skills, particularly amongst relatives and informal carers.

In the case of MND detailed technical actions in relation to problems are not only a notable feature of daily management procedures, they may become the essence of that management. For example, in relation to difficulties in swallowing, which may be an early and very troubling symptom of the bulbar form of the disease, but which often becomes a major symptom of many forms of MND/ALS as they progress, the technical knowledge acquired by relatives can be – in everyday terms – extraordinary. Judith recounts, almost by rote, the detailed knowledge she felt she had to acquire of the swallowing process to assist her elderly husband with MND/ALS, who has since died. This technical analysis, she argues, is necessary to understand the remedy – instantly – to a range of major problems which can result from a failure to swallow efficiently:

> The swallow is a very complex event; it demands precise coordination and timing of several different muscle groups. Our teeth

chop the food into a paste, the tongue forms the paste into a ball of food and sends it back into the throat. When the ball of food hits the tonsil area it triggers the swallow reflex: the larynx is elevated to hide just under the base of the tongue and the epiglottis falls over the opening into the larynx so that the airway passage is closed. The ball of food then moves into the oesophagus and, with a series of muscle squeezes and opening and closing of sphincters, the ball of food goes from the oesophagus into the stomach. The airway passage into the lungs remains clear. You can feel and watch the coordination of the elevation of the larynx by putting your hand over your Adam's apple as you swallow. If the larynx doesn't elevate quickly enough, then some of the ball of food may slip into the larynx. A good strong cough is a way of trying to get this ball of food out of the airway in order to protect the lungs. [She then notes the problems of people with MND/ALS, which may be to do with]: (a) if the tongue (which is all muscle) is weak then the ball of food isn't formed and food can slip into the throat in a disorganized manner and not trigger the reflex; (b) because of slow moving and poorly coordinated muscles, the larynx may not elevate quickly and portions of the ball of food can flow into the larynx; (c) if one doesn't have a strong, protective cough, then portions may slip through the larynx and into the lungs; (d) often clear liquids like water travel through the weakened system too quickly. Many people have more difficulty with water than thicker fluids.

This level of detailed physiological knowledge, whilst it is of course not universal in this particular form, is surprisingly widespread as, through trial and error, people with MND/ALS, and those giving them personal care, struggle to work out how to avoid alarming episodes of choking. With a condition such as MND/ALS ordinary 'non-expert' health knowledge by family members in such situations becomes increasingly of limited value, as detailed local diagnostic analysis as well as accurate management of any difficulty is immediately required, often when health care professionals are not available. At the same time, preventative strategies become crucial in relation to eating and drinking. Procedures for minimising choking are of key importance in discussions about the management of the disease between people with the disease and their relatives, as well as in discussions with health care professionals.

Some relevant procedures and 'recipes' are noted by Paul, as part of the process of exchanging a catalogue of ideas to avoid the much feared problem of choking:

1   If you are unable to chew properly, and control your food with your tongue, never start to eat any pieces of food that are large enough to block your throat.
2   Mix your food, particularly if it is dry, with a sauce of other food that will act as a lubricant, and help food slide down your throat.
3   Swallow each bite before taking the next. Never let food build up in your throat.
4   Never eat food that will mat or stick together, such as fresh bread, or sticky desserts.
5   When swallowing, concentrate and keep your chin down.
6   Learn and practice early, what to do and what not to do when you start to choke, so that later on when it happens, you won't panic. (etc.)

As we noted in Chapter 4, the understandable preoccupation with almost the slightest nuance of such problems concertinas time into a concentrated present and an anxiety-provoking immediate future. However, in MND/ALS the issue of managing swallowing and potentially associated choking difficulties is not just a cyclical task based on largely predictable, well-prepared and carefully staged eating or drinking 'events' – which may themselves last for many minutes and possibly, in very difficult situations, an hour or two – but is a continuous problem with excess and hard to manage salivation, as well as with phelgm (thickened mucus).

Indeed for some people with MND, the problem of dealing with saliva is almost the worst aspect of the disease, for frequently compounding swallowing complications – an 'internal' problem – are what are known euphemistically as 'drooling' problems, as saliva 'leaks' in a relatively uncontrolled way externally from the mouth. This latter symptom is socially as well as physically hard to manage, partly because it depicts in cultural terms a body partly out of control – as the 'inside' leaks to the 'outside'. Although saliva is usually not considered as culturally problematic and polluting as other substances, such as urine and faeces – which can in other conditions (and occasionally in MND/ALS) indicate in general terms an 'incontinent' body – the symptom is likely to be linked in the social domain to a negative view of older people identified and discussed by Mitteness and Barker (1995).

The degree to which effective control of salivation and phlegm is a pre-eminent consideration for many people with the disease, is indicated in the wide and very robust range of interventions which have been devised to reduce or control the secretions. These interventions range from local and pragmatic managerial techniques, resonating with those concerned with the consumption of food and drink, to pharmaceutical modes of control, to surgical procedures on the salivary glands, and also to radiation treatments – whose occasional and experimental use has been based on the side effects (considerably decreased salivation) of radiotherapy employed in relation to certain cancers. Geoff recounts his problems with both his salivation and what he describes as the 'dreaded mucus':

> I have found the problems I have with this dreaded mucus horrible to manage. It seems to get everywhere in my mouth, I can't seem to swallow it. I try and cough it up but I haven't really got the strength to do it. I've tried [name of several drugs] but they don't seem to work. I've heard about some surgery which might deal with my saliva problems, and recently there was a report about radiation controlling saliva – I'm not so sure about that, but if it worked, well it would be worth it.

One other person described the mucus as like constantly having 'sticky chewing gum in your mouth all the time'. Whatever she did it was there. John jokes about what others would see – and he did as well – as an embarrassingly funny situation.

> A visit to a dentist even in these modern times is no source of amusement. With all those shining instruments of torture . . . it is all a bit too much. However HUMOUR that irrepressible fun thing can often be found in the most unlikely places. With mouth wide open and suction pump working at full capacity MN goes into its act of producing what is called for the want of a better word 'rope', that resilient tough colourless saliva, that is exclusive to MN. Having capped a tooth and removing the mould the ROPE seemingly is reluctant to let go of its new found friend. It tenaciously clings all the way to the side table. The dentist endeavours to break this with an instrument but resilience prevails, and he by this time is like a fisherman with a tangle. The nurse removes the suction pipe and she too becomes embroiled

with this insidious ROPE. There seems no end to the supply and the nurse gets the giggles. Dentist also sees the humour. They are too polite to comment so I do not enlighten them, but I must smile to show off my newly acquired asset.

In all these ways the mouth, with its associated muscles, elements and functions, and its capacity to assist materials into other parts of the body, or propel them outside, becomes a centrally important part of the life of someone with MND/ALS. Increasingly, of course, detailed knowledge of the mouth of the person with MND/ALS, and its structure and functional properties, has to extend to others, as Judith's account above reveals. Thus they, as well as the person with MND/ALS, become locked into those properties. Indeed, the position is even more profoundly important than this point suggests because effective respiration, and how easily the 'breath of life' enters the body through the mouth, is also linked implicitly to how constructive and positive the management of other substances – food, drink, saliva and mucus – can be.

The danger, personally and socially speaking, in this continuing and necessary focus on life-preserving strategies by family members is not only, as Burnfield argues in relation to multiple sclerosis, that 'lovers become nurses' (Burnfield 1984), but that 'the person' at the heart of these instrumental ministrations could become lost for others in the accretion of technical tasks, as members of the family become 'body maintenance men or women'. Such a possibility is more likely in MND/ALS, not often because of the decline in cognitive capacity as in Alzheimer's disease, but because of an additional problem for many people with MND/ALS – that is a severe restriction in, or complete absence of, their 'natural' voice production. These losses lead to a very broad question, what makes us who we are to others, and at what point do we cease to be who we were?

What makes us who we are to others is a complicated issue, but it is the case that long-standing spoken, as well as bodily mannerisms and inflections, and combinations of the two, are key markers in this process, which are often severely compromised in MND/ALS. We referred in Chapter 2 to Bourdieu's (1984) notion of the 'habitus', in which recognisable techniques of the body, based on socially learnt and structured ways of doing things, form who we are. The inroads that disease, and particularly MND/ALS, makes into, first, these long-standing techniques – our mannerisms and so on – and then into how we are seen by others, is a moot point. Clearly, physical

movements in space and chronological time may be severely circumscribed, and continuing embodied possibilities of not only how, but
what is eaten and drunk, as well as many other aspects of daily life,
may be substantially changed. For Irene, her father has changed radically because of the MND in all sorts of ways:

> From this day nearly eight years ago we have seen a lot of
> changes in his physical appearance. From once a very fit man
> who played football, and a man who used to paint and decorate
> for a job as well as a hobby, there is now a man who is a shadow
> of his former self . . . It was not only his physical appearance that
> had changed it was also his temperament and how he reacted to
> once simple facts of life from a once easy going man who
> enjoyed a drink, good company and enjoyed a very good sense of
> humour there is left a man who cannot use his hands to hold a
> cup, he cannot walk as far as he used to, a sure mark of change
> that his muscles have started to deteriorate in his legs. His speech
> has slurred quite significantly, people who don't know him think
> he is drunk. This results in him becoming very frustrated as he
> cannot express his feelings or points of view in a coherent
> fashion. He has become very short tempered and has adopted
> that 'he is always right' attitude . . . So this disease has not only
> had a physical effect on how he runs his life but also mentally
> and emotionally . . . So really he is no longer the man of old,
> how everybody used to know him, but a man who has changed
> from a friendly man into a monster at times.

However, even so, most people's identities are resilient, and often
remarkably inelastic apparently to the most severe changes in their
physical persons and circumstances. For many partners – husbands
and wives – the essence of the person they knew, and still know,
remains despite the effects of the disease, indeed becomes stronger
because of it. As Peggy says about her husband:

> I admire him so much because of what he is going through. He
> doesn't complain much, and when I think of our lives together
> over all these years, and what we have meant to each other, I still
> think he's the man he was – even though he can't do so many
> things now.

The relationship of the voice and the person is a particularly
interesting issue, which Irene comments on above. Publicly, there are
few people, for example, who will have been aware of the inflections

and mannerisms of Stephen Hawking's 'natural' voice before that was effectively lost and he gained a new electronic vocal identity, which at one and the same time is now part of his person, whilst being just as obviously a generic North American electronic voice. For him to change (back?) to an avowedly middle English, Scottish, or any other kind of accent – which would be electronically and instantly possible – would reconstruct his complete identity as well as his voice. None the less, his case, and that of many others with MND/ALS, who 'speak' through many types of electronically assisted media, suggest that what anthropologists would call 'personhood', is not intrinsically bound up with a particular voice in a literal sense. To think this way is to neglect many other elements which make up what people produce and what they hear, such as the ways in which words and phrases and humour are deployed.

Technologies, as we have seen with communication technologies, as well as particular everyday social techniques play a large part in the lives of many people with MND, and perhaps even more so people who are assisting them. Technologies in the sense of non-human interventions in the lives of people with MND – ranging from drugs, to wheelchairs, to beds, to suction devices for mucus, and many others – accumulate over the course of managing the lives of persons with MND/ALS. These technologies may positively assist, or frustratingly not assist, the particular and current management task. Detailed and careful experimentation is usually the way such tasks are managed, both to find the best devices and to work out the best ways of using them in practice. Such experimentation is necessary, not only because of the particular problem of the moment, but also because of the need to meet a constantly shifting challenge of new symptoms or more problematic existing ones. Gail discusses the approach, made worse by dealing with all kinds of agencies outside the home:

> The delays, frustrations and anomalies in dealing with bureaucracy were formidable. Probably it was good for our days to be taken up with phone calls, letter writing, and devising gadgets. It allowed us to vent our fury at life on persons unknown. Every day, every week, we invented or modified something and found someone to carry out the idea. Never mind that by next month it was useless. It had served its purpose. We hadn't then realised what every handicapped person knows – that it is the very necessity which makes you the mother of invention. You may not be

able to prevent disablement; you'll be damned if you'll put up with the handicap!

All sorts of everyday equipment are dragooned into action with a bit of ingenuity and thought:

A coffee grinder works well for crushing up pills to be mixed for use in feeding. We had a small manual twist type pill crusher, but there were two problems with it: 1) there were too many pills for it to handle at a time; 2) some of the pills were coated and the coating didn't get crushed small enough to get through the feeding tube without danger of clogging. The coffee grinder solves both problems, although you just have to check with your doctor that it's OK to crush them. Some time-release medicines as well as some forms of vitamins/mineral should not be crushed!!! The coffee grinder is really very cheap.

None the less, many caring tasks are just hard labour where the physical capacities and skills of the person, as well as their constant attention, are at a premium and call upon all their reserves, especially if they are older themselves, as George was when he was managing his wife's MND/ALS:

I found at first there was a problem when she could walk a little, and she sometimes fell – or rather sank to the floor, and as she was 12 stone and although I was quite fit at 67 I found it difficult to get her up again, especially as she hated me calling for help. I therefore devised a way of doing this. I got her to sit on the floor then I put a low stool at her back and lifted her on to this by pulling her under the arms, as she still had the use of her arms she could help. I then got her onto an ordinary kitchen chair. I bought her a special high chair which helped in the early stages, but it was necessary to use a footstool to avoid restricting the leg circulation and causing pain of 'pins and needles'. At the end of her illness I did everything for her – Bathing, toilet, washing etc., but before she became too helpless I wheeled her up to the sink where she could wash up, wash herself, wash her hair and even do a small clothes wash. I used to transfer her to a tall stool for this.

This problem is compounded even more when the particular skills and knowledge acquired in undertaking these tasks are such that the person with MND/ALS only wishes to have help or support from that one person:

Gradually he was too frail to go out at all; his breathing was becoming more laboured. We had a light wheelchair on each floor. He dreaded being lifted by anyone other than me. Together we had it to a fine art. I'd wheel him from bedroom to little room next door where the steel 'filing cabinet' was, lift him on to the seat, belt him up and run downstairs to be in the sittingroom below as the lift appeared. Then into the second chair and finally decant him on to the sofa where he remained propped up by all his self-designed foam cushions until it was time to reverse the whole procedure at night. Only on one occasion did we fail and he ended up on his back on the carpet. He smilingly thanked the policeman neighbour who responded to our call for help, but no, we could manage the rest ourselves. The following night, having got him to bed without problems, he smiled up at me, 'I didn't let you down tonight, did I!'

DYING WITH MND/ALS

Thinking about death and dying, and even more mentioning or discussing death, are difficult things to do in most social settings in Western cultures. As Shilling notes:

The prospect of death cannot be contained easily within such a context [where the space occupied by religion and the sacred has shrunk, and where youth and the future are prized more than prosperity] because it represents no future in a culture orientated to futures.

(1993: 193)

In part, to quote Shilling again, this may be because:

The reduction of the scope of the sacred from the wider cosmos to the area of individual existence mirrors the transference of the significance of the death from the social body to the individual body. This general privatisation of meaning and experience leaves embodied individuals alone with the difficult task of constructing and maintaining values to guide them through life and death.

(1993: 196)

As Baumann (1992) comments (quoted in Shilling (1993)):

People find it difficult to know what to say to a dying person partly because they have no further use for the language of survival.

(Shilling 1993: 196)

In a sense, there are three sets of issues involved in dealing with the knowledge of imminent death: the first is on what basis the knowledge is available, or can be ascertained, and who has that knowledge; the second is managing that knowledge oneself, and the third is managing the knowledge in relation to others, particularly when their knowledge base about the situation is unclear. These kinds of issues are not easy to deal with, especially in the context of a close and continuing – minute-by-minute – relationship with, and maintenance of, the dying person. Some people – usually relatives – have a very clear view of their position on these matters, a position which is then often implicitly followed by the doctor. After indicating earlier that he had firmly decided from the beginning not to tell his wife she had a terminal illness, Mark recounts her last few hours. It appears, however, that she knew what was happening, and indeed may well have known all along, and he wanted the doctor at that point to inform his wife – but the doctor had his own opaque way of handling the situation:

Her health had remained fairly stable for some weeks before and there was no evidence of nor reason to anticipate a decline until just before her death. Hence, the end came quite swiftly. In the evening . . . at about seven o'clock when she was about to have her supper, she developed a high temperature, very suddenly and unexpectedly, something which had never happened previously. It was accompanied by a very flushed appearance . . . I thought that she was about to die . . . It was obvious that she must take nourishment of some sort [after not eating that day] . . . [therefore] I decided that the doctor should be called . . . The doctor came . . . he was unsuccessful [in undertaking tube feeding]. I told him [the doctor] . . . we did not want her to go into hospital . . . She then turned to the doctor and asked him 'Am I going to die, doctor?' He evaded the question by talking of the need to take some form of sustenance to maintain life. She again asked him 'Am I going to die?' I said gently to the doctor 'She wants an answer, doctor.' Again he would not answer directly but referred to an IRA hunger-strike which was then going on in Belfast and said 'The IRA hunger-strikers manage to go many days without food.' He would say no more than that. When the doctor had left, she . . . turned to me and said with the ghost of a smile 'To think that I should have to die like the IRA' . . . she had a surprisingly restful night . . . our son and daughters [who were staying with us] were round her bedside the early morning holding her hands . . . She ceased breathing at about 9 a.m. I asked my son to confirm that she had died.

For others the position is almost reversed for, from well before the time of death, the person with MND/ALS is aware not only of the likely trajectory of their disease, but believe they are aware of their specific point on that trajectory. Thus they may be anxious, and perhaps even insistent, on discussions about issues of death and dying in the face of the reluctance of a partner or relative to engage in such debates. Such discussions can be very demanding, especially if they involve ethically and personally even more troubling issues such as the possibility of robust means of prolonging life, or euthanasia. It is as though the situation of managing the physical consequences of the physical decline of MND/ALS is more than enough to bear for relatives, without being reminded by the person with the disease about both their sense of the injustice of it all, and that they find it difficult or impossible to bear. Karen's attempts to manage the increasingly demanding physical and functional needs of her mother were compounded by her mother's commentary on her own plight, and the ways in which her reflections raised and compounded old family wounds. In addition, it made Karen think about her own future:

I had to look after my mother, as she progressively became weaker, and her movements were affected. She had to be lifted up out of the chair, and I had to make the food for her, though she could feed herself albeit with a jerky movement of her arm. Regrettably my brother and his wife, who lived elsewhere did not take much interest in helping . . . as there had been arguments and disagreements in the family over the years – in fact it seemed as if my brother's wife . . . was quite happy at what had befallen my mother . . . My mother, on the other hand blamed her disease on her daughter in law . . . The disease carried on its remorseless course – and it was very unpleasant to see this sight every day for me, also it was very unpleasant for my mother to feel herself getting weaker and find that her movements were becoming impaired – she could not understand what had happened and kept saying 'Why has God punished me?' My mother . . . had been a very religious person all her life . . . her mother had taught her, 'Think of other people – help others, and God will reward you.' During the course of the disease she said to me 'Where is God?' She also said 'Is this my reward?' and [I wondered even whether] perhaps I would get a similar 'reward' as in some respects I was like her. She prayed for a cure . . . but the disease got gradually worse . . . [and] later she wanted euthanasia and asked me to give her poison. If she could have got up [then] she would have taken poison.

Others may find a possible answer precisely where Karen and her mother can find only an impossible question. Michael has taken a profoundly philosophical view of his position with the disease as he contemplates death:

there is the towering thought. The number of my days is known not to myself but to God. I have always been religious to an extent as has been my wife. This has turned into a great but complex support. Cardinal Newman distinguished between notional and real assent. The former is the agreement we give to an intellectual, scientific or logical proposition. Real assent results from what we know in our guts . . . the burning conviction which moves us to action. My assent to my situation was, I realised a month ago, only notional when I woke in the night terrified because I realised that I could well be totally paralysed. The terror and despair lay around me like an impenetrable black blanket. I prayed and was succoured. I don't think I am afraid of death but certainly [I am afraid of] the process of decay and dying. I am conscious of the support of friends and organisations. But I must change from a life which is intensely independent concerned with physical things to a life which, whatever its length, is going to be largely mental, spiritual and totally dependent upon others. How will I stand it? Prayer helps. But the test of real assent is still to come. Luckily I am naturally an optimist.

Of course one of the problems about discussing dying and death is that it may not be clear, particularly to a wife or husband, son or daughter, whether the person with MND not only knows about the situation but wishes to discuss it. Pat shares her view about this issue:

my husband has been having an increasingly difficult time

dealing with my illness and during one of those painful heart to heart talks that are part of dealing with MND, he reluctantly shared those feelings with me. He said he didn't want to talk about those feelings [about dying and its consequences] because he thought it would sound as if he were impatiently waiting for me to die and stop messing up his life. He thought that it would upset me to hear that he thought about the things he would be able to do when I was gone. He was shocked when I told him how relieved I was to hear it! His refusal to discuss the future at all had me fearing that he simply couldn't see that there was a light at the end of the tunnel for him. That discussion eased my worries about him and eased his guilty feelings about thinking that life will be easier when I'm gone. Maybe it is basic, but everyone needs to hear that it is OK to see a light at the end of the tunnel.

These accounts in their various ways appear to raise the issue of not so much the fact of death, but the manner and timing of death. Slater argues from his review:

it is the process of dying that concerns older people more than death itself.

(1995: 141)

Such a view has been echoed in many studies elsewhere (for example, Aries 1981; Williams 1990; Jefferys 1996). However, we have argued earlier MND/ALS has to be considered in the context of not only chronological life (how old people are), but on the meanings attributed to times of life or points in the life course. Without being over precise about the boundary between the two, it is the case in MND/ALS that there is a distinction between those people, predominantly younger (or younger old), who consider the prospect of death itself as absolutely unacceptable 'at their time of life', and other people who are predominantly older who are exceedingly anxious – as are often their relatives – about the mode of dying, rather than the fact of dying. None the less, for all, the mode of dying is of the utmost importance. To rephrase the issue, people with MND/ALS, and even more so their relatives, are looking as the disease advances for a 'good death' if the disease cannot be prevented from progressing. This is a very problematic issue in an age of individualism for, as Shilling notes:

[even if] the subjective deferral of death can be sought in

investing meaning and hope in a loved one . . . the loved one is another mortal creature whose very existence provides regular reminders of bodily fragility and mortality . . . [especially in relation to] ageing bodies . . . [and further modernity has] left people alone with their bodies in the face of death.

(1993: 193)

What a 'good death' is, is itself a matter of debate. Furthermore, the translation from a cosmic to an individualistically based approach to death means that pre-existing and widely accepted public rituals of dying have become fractured, so that to a large extent individuals are compelled to construct their own ways of managing this process, synthesising them with available ideas, images and structures. In response to this situation, the creation of hospices is one of the latest attempts to provide a more formalised, proper and acceptable way of dying, of which an increasing number of people with MND/ALS are taking advantage. In part, a 'good death' is *what is not* present leading up to the point of death, and that is pain and suffering – in the broadest sense of the word – as well as the dying and death being in an inappropriate place, at an inappropriate time, and with inappropriate people. In part, it is what is present, both in the form of appropriate places, time and people, but also a sense of the roundedness of life, the completing of an agenda, in which social and personal hurts are reconciled as far as possible, final goodbyes are said, and the transition from life to death is accomplished peacefully in every sense of that word. Just stating these broad points, and considering them in the context of the accounts above, suggests the realisation of a 'good death' is a rather complicated process. Family members face tremendously difficult dilemmas and decisions in this context.

In some cases, such as Trisha's, she felt she had to hand over the care of her husband in his final hours to the hospital, but thought that in the circumstances his dying went well, and contrary to other accounts the medical and other staff managed him with skill, although she was not present at the moment of death:

Five days later [after we moved to our new bungalow] he became very ill. He held his hand to his ear telling me to phone the doctor. I dialled 999. In Accident and Emergency I tried to explain he was Motor Neurone. They must have laid him flat, the alarm bells were ringing, I knew they were resuscitating him. He was taken into Intensive Care, his brain still active writing on his note pad 'what happened'. They were marvellous with him. He was later transferred, he was not happy. I asked for cot sides and an extra pillow. He was cross with me for the very first time, he wrote on his pad my legs are useless because I did not have enough exercise. I felt very sad there was nothing more I could do for him. I had looked after him with tender loving care. The next morning I had a call to the hospital his pulse was very weak, I fled down the corridor but was too late to be with him at the end, but he looked so peaceful.

In Penny's situation after having nursed her mother for many years she, Penny:

carried on until they finally forcibly took her [mother] – to [name of hospital] – where I visited her. She was finally completely paralysed, unable to move a muscle, and given oxygen, plus being specially fed – it was extremely distressing to see. I could still make out a few words, though no one else could. On one visit I told her I wished I had accomplished more in life but my mother, who was just lying there, motioned to my hand with her eyes and kissed my hand – later I made out she wanted me to leave. Some time later I had a phone call to say she was 'deteriorating', and then she died.

To some this might seem a slightly unsatisfactory way to end the relationship in life between mother and daughter, but as Penny indicates she was herself very distressed by her mother's condition and may have preferred to remember her as she was, rather than in an alien medical environment. For other people with MND, keeping up appearances in the face of tremendous odds is what has made them who they are both to their relatives and to other staff. Kirsty talks about her husband in his final couple of days:

One morning he was being very weak, and I asked if we could have a visit [from the GP]. The Doctor examined him – fully dressed, shaved and every last hair in place by his own wish – and said 'I think you should have a day or two upstairs in bed. Just to rest a little, you know.' 'I'M NOT AN INVALID' he whispered in what would have been a shout. Downstairs, the Doctor said to me he really needed to be admitted to hospital. He hadn't got very long. I said, no, I didn't want his life prolonged by the carrying out of miserable procedures and resustications [sic] and I would rather get more nursing help if I couldn't manage alone.

That night, I had for the first time a night nurse, a very young girl lacking in confidence. I kept getting up to see if all were well. Geoff seemed to be hallucinating. In the morning he was awake and lucid. 'I missed you terribly,' he said. It made me feel a swine. He asked for breakfast and again insisted on being washed and dressed, but was then content to remain lying on the bed. The lovely little nurse from the practice popped in. 'I'll put your pyjamas on' she said, 'you'll be more comfortable.' He glared at her, 'NOT AN INVALID' he mouthed. That was about the last thing he said. During the afternoon he lapsed into unconsciousness and at eight in the evening, so very gently, his breathing faded away.

For Vivian and his wife, managing his mother at home until the end proved impossible. The progression in her MND/ALS was relatively quick and for three months after her diagnosis his wife:

was at home ... where I attempted to look after her [his mother] and assist her, but following a further visit to the hospital it was arranged for her to go to the [name of hospice] where she remained until she died. I brought her home every weekend but by this time all walking ability had gone and her speech was very difficult, also she had major eating problems – only sloppy food and soups being possible. Her intelligence, memory and the desire to look feminine remained with her to the end – in fact by use of letto cards ... we were able to put down on paper a short poem, based on her life, that she had 'written' whilst at the hospice. This was subsequently published in the hospice report after her death.

It appears for Vivian (and perhaps his wife) that his mother's situation was handled as well as it could have been given other constraints, and that she had, from their point of view, as good a death as she reasonably could have done in a hospice setting.

Although in a number of these accounts relatives were not present at the death of the person with MND, it is clear that for others being present at the death of a close relative is an important – one might say a vital – social and personal act. For as Rubinstein argues:

The experience of death is ... decreasingly a community or a congregational event and instead the business of a diffusely defined family, a social network or 'the immediate family'.

(1995: 257)

It is the family presence which in many ways cements the *rite de passage* from life to death, as in Sandra's account of her mother's death:

[Following the diagnosis] we had expected a year or so of further deterioration . . . and were planning that she would move to a hospice, but not for the moment . . . thus . . . the end took us by surprise. On that morning, my husband and I were surprised to receive a buzzer call during our breakfast [from a bedroom in their house where her mother and father were living]. Mum had somehow roused Dad, and he thought she needed the commode. Mum could no longer tell us if this was so – and we quickly realised she was not communicating at all, even with her eyes. However, my husband and I lifted Mum in the usual way, but before my husband could withdraw from the room we could see her head falling to one side – she could no longer support it. We lifted her gently back to bed, & I immediately called out a doctor. A Doctor came within minutes, and he told us at once that Mum was in a coma. Dad and I had to leave the room, presumably while he tried to rouse her, but he shortly rejoined us to tell us the end was now very near. Dad could not accept this. He sat & read a letter from Mum's (other) sister to Mum in case she could still hear. My husband had already rung my mother's sister and then we were all here . . . but Mum did not regain consciousness. In retrospect, we found comfort in the fact that Mum was spared even further deterioration (and that Dad was spared this, too) and a move into hospital or hospice.

CHOICES ABOUT THE END OF LIFE

It is often assumed that the point at which life ends is both clear, and 'natural', and that in those senses death is a self-evident state. It has also been assumed as a corollary that the range of choices around the event, and particularly the timing of death are limited, both by virtue of their technical possibility, and by virtue of their ethical, social and personal consequences. In recent years, however, the point at which people with MND/ALS both do die, and even more, should die, and through what means, has become a matter of increasingly vigorous and contentious discussion. This is also part of a much wider debate on several key issues, particularly on the criteria by which death is established, and – even if such criteria can be agreed – about the range of ways in which that point can be controlled medically, technologically or personally through explicit choice. In other words, both the point of death and the means by which it occurs is a highly contested area.

A number of recent papers have challengingly documented the ways in which criteria for death have been subject to change and redefinition both medically and culturally. Perhaps the most significant development in the Western world in recent years in attempting to specify when death occurs has been that related to the idea of brain death. Giacomini has examined the ambitious attempt by a committee of medical staff at Harvard University in 1968 to establish criteria for brain death, and whilst the committee did not establish undisputed criteria for brain death, they did establish it as a technical 'fact':

> [and that] . . . brain death had standard, 'objective' clinical features. The question became not, what 'means' death to family, clergy, caretakers or others involved with a patient . . . but what 'is' death in objectively measurable terms.
>
> (1997: 1479)

Of particular importance for people with MND/ALS was the fact that the role of ventilators (to mechanically assist breathing) were not considered at this time in relation to (preventing) brain death. For indeed in North America there has been over recent years a considerable – a remarkable – increase in the numbers of people with very advanced disease who are now using assisted breathing techniques, or are considering doing so (Mitsumoto and Norris 1994). Whilst the use of these techniques themselves is not designed in the case of MND/ALS to remedy or assist already damaged brains, in very advanced cases of the disease where they supplement and then replace 'natural' respiration, death would be speedy without them. The length of time for which continuous mechanical ventilation can keep people with MND/ALS alive beyond where they would otherwise have died is still under investigation (and development). It appears to hinge largely on the quality of the huge amount of ancillary care which is required to maintain the person on the ventilator. However, several years of life are plainly possible.

It is a particularly interesting phenomenon that the other country where ventilators have been relatively widely used for people with MND/ALS is Japan, where criteria for death are completely different from those in North America. After noting that there has been a complete rejection of brain death criteria in Japan, Lock indicates that:

> efforts to assign death scientifically to a measurable point in time are [also] often rejected outright. Death is understood as a social event by the majority, amongst whom clinicians are included. Both the biological and cognitive status of the patient is assigned secondary importance.
>
> (1996: 577)

In Japan, therefore, the issue of possible ventilation for people with MND/ALS fits more neatly into cultural understandings which would allow, perhaps even welcome, such a possibility. However in Britain, and a number of other countries outside North America and Japan, there appears to have been a tacit agreement amongst senior health care staff, particularly neurologists, that assisted breathing equipment of such a complete and continuous kind, which would do more than relieve discomfort and suffering, would not be supported in the case of MND/ALS. As far as is known, there are very few, if any, people with MND/ALS using such equipment in Britain. Thus, in effect the choices available on a routine or regular basis for people with MND/ALS in Britain and much of Europe would not include this possibility. The arguments for such a restriction on what could be described as a long-term palliative technique, are that indeed it almost heroically prolongs life whilst the neurological status of the person is still declining; the quality of life for the user of such equipment would be (assumed to be) very poor; the financial costs – to the person, their family or private or public sources – would be astronomical and not be counterbalanced by corresponding benefits; the equation for social and personal costs would be even less viable, and the ethical standing of recommending such a course of action is problematic. However, despite these huge caveats, the totally different (medical) practices in this respect in different parts of the world in relation to very advanced cases of MND/ALS do raise major ethical and related questions, particularly about patient autonomy and choice.

It is tempting to argue – as we have throughout this text – that the social and demographic features of those with MND/ALS, particularly their usually (relatively) advanced age on diagnosis, has placed them in the category of older patients whose choices (not just in respect of ventilators to prolong life) on some potential ameliorative strategies are relatively restricted (Jefferys 1996). In other words, there is an ethical issue which deserves further exploration about the basis on which older people with a range of neurological conditions receive some medical interventions and not others.

This issue of using mechanical means to prolong life is one about which some people with MND/ALS – particularly in North America and Japan – feel strongly and positively, and about which they feel they should have a choice. On the other hand, perhaps many more people with MND/ALS in Britain and Europe, as well as in North America and the rest of the world, feel just as strongly that a choice to consider ending (rather than extending) their life with the disease should both be able to be discussed and, in appropriate circumstances, be able to be acted upon. In some of the accounts of people with MND/ALS already explored in this chapter, and in many more which have been drawn upon, the possibility of making such a choice to end life forms part both of their narrative of the disease, as well as that of a number of those caring for them. This issue of choice about the time to die is usually discussed as 'euthanasia'. Caddell and Newton, in their study of American attitudes towards the physician's role in euthanasia, argue for a clear distinction to be made between active (intentional killing) and passive (letting die) forms of euthanasia. In their terms:

> active euthanasia–[is]–any treatment *by a physician* [authors' emphasis] with the intent of hastening the death of another human being who is terminally ill and in severe pain or distress with the motive of relieving that person from great suffering.

And:

> suicide–[is]–the terminal patient taking steps to end their own life independent of a physician's assistance for the purpose of shortening their suffering.

> (1995: 1472)

Placing together the findings of the work of Seale *et al.* in Britain (1997) and that of Caddell and Newton (1995) in the United States in respect of what the latter describe as active euthanasia, it appears that there is both a high level of public support for such euthanasia and that support is growing. Thus, it seems likely that people with MND/ALS in the future, as well as those with other terminal conditions, will not only be more willing to discuss such issues, but may well take a more robust approach to them. Recent court cases in Britain by people with MND/ALS seeking clarification of, as well as challenging, the legal position on physician-assisted death, well-publicised (and televised) cases of euthanasia from Europe, as well as other vigorous public debates involving people with MND, also suggest that this issue will remain a high-profile one, not only for particular individuals, but also for collective views and judgements.

The conventional medical view in Britain and North America about what is described above as active euthanasia is decidedly different from those described in these two recent analyses, and also that indicated from surveys of public opinion. By and large, it can be described as one which acknowledges the difficulties raised by living with terminal illness, but is based on the view that most requests for active euthanasia arise through poor symptom and, particularly, pain control. If that control is achieved then there should be no good reason for a request for active euthanasia, or acceding to such a request. The difficulty with this position, even if it proves to be the case, is that it does ground choice in relation to this very fundamental decision on a different basis to that on any other medical procedure. It reinserts authority in the place of autonomy and 'choice'.

A bioethical analysis of the position also raises a complex set of problems. As Cole and Holstein (1996) point out, the basis of decision-making in medicine in many industrialised societies is 'informed consent'. The problem is that, in principle, this is a satisfactory procedure, while in practice it is often flawed, particularly in the way that it is often procedurally conceived – as a single one-off (informed) agreement between physician and patient. A morally, more satisfactory, way of considering informed consent, on many of the difficult medical decisions that affect people with MND, is to argue for it:

> as part of an ongoing, open-ended conversation in which patient, physician, other providers, and family members reach a provisional consensus about care.
>
> (ibid.: 482)

And further, to see that communal approach as:

> Negotiation . . . when no interest trumps all others and when love and compassion confront autonomy.
>
> (ibid.: 483)

Such an approach seems sensible, but it seems most sensible well in advance of the problems to which the informed consent occurs. What are collectively known as 'advance directives' – formal, signed and witnessed statements – by the person with MND/ALS are one way of seeking to pre-empt and manage future problematic situations:

> [They] allow individuals in advance of incapacitation to decide how they wish to be treated and who would make decisions.
>
> (ibid.: 483)

They are more helpful in indicating the limits to what individuals wish done to them (in the way of procedures, or resuscitation, and so on) rather than indicating that 'everything should be done'. The latter is difficult for others (including physicians) to interpret. Of course, by their existence, they may inhibit discussion at the time of the problem about other options. On the other hand, if they do not exist there may be problems, in certain circumstances, in deciding what the preferred option of the person with MND/ALS might be. In this respect, immediate family judgements and advice may be critical, and indeed may be the only source of advice based on intimate knowledge of the person that a doctor may have available. However, there is a considerable body of research which indicates that there may be substantial discrepancies on occasion between family views and that of the person concerned as to what their wishes might be (Pearlman *et al.* 1992; Seckler *et al.* 1991).

However, despite these potential difficulties between family members and the person concerned over what their wishes might be, Cole and Holstein note that:

> the moral world inhabited by most older individuals is not adequately captured in a theory-driven bioethics that relies on a 'free agent' view of the self . . . [thus] the possibilities for actual as opposed to ideal autonomy . . . depend on social and cultural contexts in which self can be expressed.
>
> (1995: 492)

In this context, the major difficulty with many of the most problematic decisions about the lives of people with MND/ALS is that whatever decision might be preferred by the person with the disease – particularly to prolong or to shorten life – it almost certainly involves others in a major way in its implementation and consequences. These others are family members, as well as doctors and other health care professionals. There is a need, as Cole and Holstein (1996) persuasively argue, for a reconsideration of the collective moral basis on which such decisions may be built.

Chapter 7

The suffering of people with motor neurone disease and the rationality of scientific medicine

THE WORLD OF SUFFERING AND THE WORLD OF RATIONALITY

We have argued throughout this book that in dissecting the experiences of people with MND/ALS we are considering two worlds. One world is a world of suffering. It is a world of people with the disease and their relatives in which both have to manage daily life, not only dealing with the major functional, social and personal problems that the condition brings, but also seeking to understand its meaning – to discover a purpose for their suffering and thereby reducing their existential uncertainty (Adamson 1997). The other world is a world of rationality. It is a world built on the application of technical knowledge, acquired predominantly through a scientific – a rational – approach to information; in short, it is the world of scientific medicine. Indeed, a main part of the narrative of this book is the story of people with the disease and their relatives seeking help from the world of scientific medicine, usually through its clinical manifestations, to enable them to manage this malevolent intervention which has befallen their lives. The nature of the relationship between these two worlds, and indeed between what could be argued to be their major paradigms, suffering and rationality, is in many ways at the heart of making sense of MND/ALS.

Byron Good (1994) extensively explores the relationship between these two worlds. Good argues, in common with many others in recent times, that there is a significant epistemological disjunction (or a difference in ways of knowing the world) between scientific medicine and what he calls 'local moral worlds of suffering'. More particularly, he indicates that the pervasiveness of rationality at the core of scientific medicine is dangerously colonising the more meaningful aspects of human existence. In particular, there is an attempt to incorporate (or, to put it more bluntly, take over) many of those aspects of life into a scientific framework to which they do not belong, and in relation to whose rational approach they cannot be understood. Thus fundamentally, he argues, it is the role of social scientists, and particularly medical anthropologists, to review critically, and indeed to challenge, this view of medicine and medical activity. This task is not only difficult because of the existing hold of such a view within the domain of contemporary medicine, but because the reach of this rationality is becoming broader and penetrating an even larger domain of human existence, not only through doctors and their activities, but through many associated professions whose basic approach employs a similar framework and set of methods.

In the light of this argument, as we have demonstrated, many kinds of questions that people with MND/ALS ask about their situation are not easily answered by reference to scientific medicine, as indeed they are not when people with other serious conditions ask them. Many such questions relate to issues of how and why they have been faced with this additional burden in their lives and raise, as Good suggests, predominantly moral issues, such as those of personal justice, of equity, of their capacity for autonomy and personal choice, of the moral basis of suffering, and of the relationship between their pasts, presents and futures. In this process, questions also relate in a complicated way to social and cultural issues about people's relationships to their families, friends and, collectively, to other people, and about their relationship to the natural and supernatural worlds, and in particular to their religious beliefs and understandings. Fran poses some (scientifically) unanswerable questions stemming from living with her husband and his MND/ALS:

> I ask myself all the time why did this disease have to come to us. We are just an ordinary family. We have lived as good a life as we could – I know we've had our problems, but then doesn't everybody? I can't understand how somebody could suffer so, it's not so much that he's in pain, but just to see him sliding away as the disease gets hold of him. What kind of world is this? Nobody deserves this to happen to them.

Such questions arise particularly in relation to lives that were once known very differently. It is not only wives or husbands who have to struggle with these questions in relation to a partner that they knew with different and far more robust physical capacities. For sons or daughters, brothers and sisters, and other relatives, it can be just as painful a process of reflection. For sons and daughters, in particular, the transition wrought rapidly by MND/ALS on a once powerful parent to an almost completely physically incapacitated person is particularly hard to bear. This is both an issue of a major loss of functional skills, but perhaps even more important a rapid, and often unexpected, change in dependency – the child has to become a parent to their parent. Although, in the course of generational transitions and ageing processes, such a change occurs regularly amongst others, it appears to be the rapidity as well as the explicit ways in which this issue is exposed by the particular drastic effects of the disease – often on a combination of mobility, eating, drinking, and voice-based communication, together with an accelerated death – that highlights this dramatic personal and social change. For Lionel this did indeed raise moral problems about his mother's MND/ALS which he found difficult to raise and impossible to answer:

It was extremely saddening to have seen the illness and afterwards I felt very depressed indeed; and I puzzled over the illness – I thought to myself money and material things are not the most important in life but health is more important – I also thought how strange is this life and uncertain – you never know what may hit you – an illness can suddenly come on – I live with the thought that some illness could hit me at any time – Parkinsons Disease, Cancer, Heart Disease – just a question of time when one of these can hit anyone and the doctors discover their unwelcome news. No one can escape the inevitable outcome of our lives. It is almost as if the doctors are waiting at the hospital for all of us – there life begins and often ends too, all we can do is to hope for a better world later – a world beyond the grave. My mother went through a terrible suffering and I suffered along with her, I kept wondering through the illness what it was that happened to her? Why it happened to her, a person who loved to be active and I tried to understand what had happened – and to have my own theory. I read medical books and so on – I kept thinking about what happened during the illness and after she died.

It might be tempting to argue that the role of scientific medicine be less than it is in the management of MND/ALS. However, this is plainly not likely to be the case, as indeed largely through the pressure of organised groups of people with MND/ALS (particularly the major voluntary national associations), and through a range of other factors, there has been an exponential growth of scientific interest in the possible causes and treatments for MND/ALS in recent years, as well as a very considerable growth in clinical centres assisting in its management.

The effects of this scientific explosion of activity are all the more striking when it is realised the extent to which previously older people in Western societies – of whom many people with MND/ALS and their relatives are a part – have largely remained outside the cutting edge of science-based medical classifications and the therapeutic zeal of its practitioners (Jefferys 1996). Although generic 'old age' has long since ceased to be a viable pigeon-hole into which those who die late in life were medically placed, the resonances of the previous widespread use of taxonomies employing notions of death as being from 'old age', as well as ideas that older people were beyond the range of many science-based medical interventions, still colour our understanding and relatively minimal expectations – even if we have great hopes – of scientific medicine at this time of life.

THE INTERVENTION OF SCIENTIFIC MEDICINE AT OLDER AGES AND ITS IMPLICATIONS FOR PEOPLE WITH MND/ALS

For many social analysts, the great increase in medical interventions amongst older people is not necessarily considered to be beneficial – contrary to the forceful advocacy of further involvement with medical science by the major voluntary national associations concerned with MND/ALS. In this respect, the breadth as well as the rapidity of recent changes in the intervention of scientific medicine at older ages has been of substantial concern to some. Illustrating this approach, Kaufman (1994), in her study of the relationship of science-based medicine to older people, describes how relatively new procedures centred on comprehensive geriatric assessment are expanding the practice of medicine beyond conventional disease categories. Using the idea of 'risk', particularly centring on functional problems which may occur given certain life styles – and of course occur in any case with a vengeance in MND/ALS – such assessments are now being used to assess and monitor many, even the majority, of older people, whether or not they have a significant disease. Thus, the everyday world of even the currently healthy old is being made a part of medical practice. These procedures, she argues, through their potential pervasiveness, are implicitly pulling many older people into a medical framework from what would otherwise be a life relatively free of such an intervention.

Kaufman's analysis can be taken – as indeed it is in large part – as a straightforward criticism about the extension of the medical enterprise to yet another group who would otherwise be left to carry on their lives in their own way outside of the unhelpful and rational world of medicine. In particular, she feels that such medical interventions amongst the relatively healthy old bypass important questions about human experience, as well as human suffering, which figure so large for people at older ages.

However, a fundamentally good case can be made which challenges the arguments of both Good and Kaufman, and shows that far from losing out from the intervention of science-based medicine in their lives, people with MND and their relatives gain from it in major, and sometimes unexpected, ways. Thus, whilst Kaufman and Good argue in their different ways that being centrally involved with the world of scientific medicine undermines and discounts the local moral worlds of suffering in which people with MND/ALS and other serious conditions live, we argue that these two worlds can be, and often are, supportive of each other.

The reason why people with MND/ALS gain from a central role for scientific medicine is the generally uncomfortable and marginal status most older people in Western societies have to the mainstream values of those societies, as well to the mainstream values of (curative) medicine. There is often a problematic elision by medical others about such older people, between their ageing, their potential and often increasing sickness, and ultimately their death, which in effect relegates them to a world of palliative care. A similar kind of disengagement to that seen in removal from the world of paid employment might be argued to occur for many older people as they are centrifugally flung out from the curative core of biomedicine to its palliative periphery.

Thus the 'gain' we are discussing, in relation to the major role for scientific medicine, is not one which may seem immediately obvious to people with the disease. For it is not that scientific medicine has produced, or indeed will produce, an early cure for MND/ALS, although some incremental progress is being made along these lines.

The 'gain' is to do with now being part of that mainstream world of medicine from which other older people have *de facto* been excluded – and in that sense becoming again part of the mainstream, rather than being still on the periphery of Western life. Therefore, people with MND/ALS can be considered now part of the world of scientific medicine with a curative thrust, not just a palliative approach to the disease.

Whilst at present the major medical support for people with MND is still of a palliative or symptomatic kind, the hope of a cure is always a component of this burgeoning scientific enterprise. Indeed, William's wife, part of whose account illustrated the arguments in Chapter 4, noted how William was one of the founding members of the MNDA in Britain precisely because there appeared to be no major scientific or medical interest in the disease at the time he was diagnosed with it. He had felt that the only way to gain recognition, not only for the disease, but more particularly for the people who were diagnosed with it, was to found an association with others to generate more scientific research into the condition. It is indeed remarkable how, over a period of a few years, such a significant body of scientific research into MND is now underway with all its organisational, professional and financial corollaries.

Therefore, whilst Kaufman and Good seem to suggest that control and individual autonomy may be surrendered by people who come into contact with scientific medicine, in the case of MND/ALS some of that control may be regained. This is, in part, to do with now not being 'just another' older person who has increasing functional problems and who is gradually slipping towards death, but with being a person with a diagnosed and named, although fatal, disease in relation to which there is considerable expert scientific effort invested in finding a cure. Moreover, this expertise is not in geriatrics and in geriatric care with its generic responsibility for all conditions in older people, it is in the medically and scientifically prestigious field of neurology. Although many conditions with which neurologists deal are present amongst older people, their role for various historic reasons has transcended and overcome the generally lower scientific status awarded to those with generic responsibilities for particular kinds of patients, rather than particular kinds of disease. Indeed, their own prestige has been helpful in importing older people into a more demographically egalitarian position in relation to medical care – that is, they are not so much an older person with a problem, they are a case of a disease with a range of impressive signs and symptoms (from the point of view of scientific medicine in general, and neurology in particular).

That is, a disease is a disease – whether of the young or of the old; thus, in a special sense, all diseases are considered within that rationality. This argument is that the common framework arising from the demographic decontextualising of MND/ALS (they are not old, they have a disease) allows both the 'victims' of this disease – motor neurone disease – and their biomedical diagnosticians and potential therapists to operate in a similar, perhaps almost in the same, framework. People with MND are increasingly seen biomedically, and many see themselves as no longer the relatively passive objects of a lengthy ageing process, but as the active subjects of a dramatic and fatal disease in which instrumental attention to the redress of its effects is part of the agenda of both parties. It becomes both an ordinary disease by virtue of it being something which can be placed in the lexicon of all other diseases, and of course an extraordinary one by virtue of its effects. As Sandra says:

> It helps to know that there is so much research going on to find a cure for MND, and all those scientists are trying as hard as they can. I never want anyone else to suffer like my husband did. I know the answer didn't come in time for him, but now we know what it is and what we are up against, I will do all I can to help the doctors and scientists.

It may be, therefore, that whilst the local worlds of suffering, which people with MND/ALS and their relatives endure and try and make sense of, are very different from the approach of the rational world of scientific medicine to the disease, their local suffering can be assisted by that different world. It helps, even in a small way, to know that MND/ALS is a 'real' disease, not just a major functional problem of older people only considered for modest palliative care, and that there is a very large scientific enterprise working its way towards a cure – no matter how far away that may be. The suffering is still there in a major way, as the accounts throughout this text demonstrate, and there are many questions which cannot, and will never be, answered by or through scientific medicine, but the presence of that rationality and the scientific part of the medical enterprise is a sign that the MND/ALS is treated as a very serious proposition to be addressed in the mainstream of social and medical life.

References

Adamson, C. (1997) 'Existential and clinical uncertainty in the medical encounter: an idiographic account of an illness trajectory defined by Inflammatory Bowel Disease and Avascular Necrosis', *Sociology of Health and Illness* 19(2): 133–59.

Age Concern (1992) *Dependence: The Ultimate Fear*, London: Age Concern.

ALS Society of Canada (1994) *Resources for Health Care Providers*, Toronto: ALS Society of Canada.

Arber, S. and Ginn, J. (eds) (1995) *Connecting Gender and Ageing*, Milton Keynes: Open University Press.

Aries, P. (1981) *The Hour of our Death*, New York: Alfred Knopf.

Arksey, H. (1994) 'Expert and lay participation in the construction of medical knowledge', *Sociology of Health and Illness* 16(4): 141–89.

Baumann, Z. (1992) *Mortality, Immortality and Other Life Strategies*, Cambridge: Polity Press.

Binstock, R. H. and George, L. K. (eds) (1996) *Handbook of Ageing and the Social Sciences*, 4th edn, San Diego: Academic Press.

Black, S. E., Blessed, G., Edwardson, J. A., and Kay, D. W. K. (1991) 'Prevalence of dementia in an ageing population', *Age and Ageing* 19: 84–90.

Bourdieu, P. (1984) *Distinction: A Social Critique of the Judgement of Taste*, London: Routledge.

Bradley, W. G. (1994) 'Amyotrophic lateral sclerosis: the diagnostic process', in H. Mitsumoto and F. H. Norris (eds), *Amyotrophic Lateral Sclerosis: A Comprehensive Guide to Management*, New York: Demos.

British Gas (1991) *British Gas Report on Attitudes to Aging*, London: British Gas.

Brown, W. A. and Mueller, P. S. (1970) 'Psychological function in individuals with amyotrophic lateral sclerosis (ALS)', *Psychosomatic Medicine* 32: 141–52.

Buckley, J., Warlow, C., Smith, P. *et al.* (1983) 'Motor neurone disease in England and Wales 1959–79', *J. Neurol. Neurosurg. Psych.* 46: 197–205.

Burnfield, A. (1984) *Multiple Sclerosis: A Personal Exploration*, London: Souvenir Press.

Bury, M. (1988) 'Meanings at risk: the experience of arthritis', in R. Anderson and M. Bury (eds) *Living with Chronic Illness: The Experience of Patients and their Families*, London: Unwin Hyman.

Caddell, D. P. and Newton, R. R. (1995) 'Euthanasia: American attitudes toward the physician's role', *Social Science and Medicine* 40(12): 1671–81.

Charcot, J. M. (1874) 'De la sclerose laterale amyotrophique', *Prog. Med.* 2: 325–7.

Christiakis, N. A. (1997) 'The ellipsis of prognosis in modern medical thought', *Social Science and Medicine* 44(3): 301–15.

Cobb, A. K. and Hamera, E. (1986) 'Illness experience in a chronic disease: ALS, *Social Science and Medicine* 23: 641–50.

Cole, T. R. and Holstein, M. (1996) 'Ethics and aging', in R. H. Binstock and L. K. George (eds), *Handbook of Ageing and the Social Sciences* 4th edn, San Diego: Academic Press.

Dugan, L. L. and Choi, D. W. (1994) 'Excitotoxity, free radicals and cell membrane changes', *Annals of Neurology* 35: 17–21.

Fleck, L. (1935) *Genesis and Developement of a Scientific Fact*, Basel: Benno Schwabe (English trans. Chicago: University of Chicago Press (1979)).

Giacomini, M. (1997) 'A change of heart and a change of mind? Technology and the redefinition of death in 1968', *Soc. Sci. Med.* 44(10): 1465–82.

Glasberg, M. R. (1994) 'Amyotrophic lateral sclerosis: unorthodox treatments', in H. Mitsumoto and F. H. Norris (eds), *Amyotrophic Lateral Sclerosis: A Comprehensive Guide to Management*, New York: Demos.

Goffman, E. (1964) *Stigma: Notes on the Management of a Spoiled Identity*, Harmondsworth: Pelican.

Good, B. (1994) *Medicine, Rationality and Experience*, Cambridge: Cambridge University Press.

Gurney, M. E., Pu, U., Chiu, A. Y. *et al.* (1994) 'Motor neurone degeneration in mice that express a human CuZn superoxide dismutase mutation', *Science* 264: 1772–5.

Harris, H. G. (1989) 'Mechanism and morality in patients' views of illness and injury', *Medical Anthropology Quarterly* 3: 3–21.

Hogg, K. E., Goldstein, L. H., and Leigh, P. N. (1994) 'The psychological impact of motor neurone disease', *Psychological Medicine* 24: 625–32.

Houpt, J. L., Gould, B. S., and Norris, F. H. (1977) 'Psychological characteristics of patients with amyotrophic lateral sclerosis (ALS)', *Psychosomatic Medicine* 39: 299–303.

Hunter, M., Robinson, I., and Neilson, S. (1993) 'The functional and psychological status of patients with MND: some implications for rehabilitation', *Disability and Rehabilitation* 15: 119–26.

Jefferys, M. (1996) 'Cultural aspects of ageing: gender and inter-generational issues', *Social Science and Medicine* 43(5): 681–7.

Jette, A. M. (1996) 'Disability trends and transitions', in R. H. Binstock and L. K. George (eds), *Handbook of Ageing and the Social Sciences* 4th edn, San Diego: Academic Press.

Kaufman, S. R. (1994) 'Old age, disease and the discourse on risk: geriatric assessment in US health care', *Medical Anthropolgy Quarterly* 8(4): 430–51.

Khabbaz, S. T. and Roos, R. P. (1994) 'Therapeutic trials in amyotrophic lateral sclerosis', in H. Mitsumoto and F. H. Norris (eds) *Amyotrophic Lateral Sclerosis: A Comprehensive Guide to Management*, New York: Demos.

Korten, A. E., Henderson, A. S., Christensen, H., Jorm, A. F., Rodgers, B., Jacomb, P., and Mackinnon, A. J. (1997) 'A prospective study of cognitive function in the elderly', *Psychological Medicine* 27: 919–30.

Kurland, L. T. and Radhakrishnan, K. (1993) 'An update of the epidemiology of Western Pacific amyotrophic lateral sclerosis', in C. A. Molgaard (ed.), *Neuroepidemiology: Theory and Method*, San Diego: Academic Press.

Lilienfeld, D. E., Chan, E., Ehland, J. *et al.* (1989) 'Rising mortality from motor neurone disease in the USA: 1962–1984', *Lancet* 35: 710–12.

Lock, M. (1996) 'Death in technological time: locating the end of meaningful life', *Medical Anthropology Quarterly* 10(4): 575–600.

McDonald, E. R. (1994) 'Psychosocial spiritual review', in H. Mitsumoto and F. H. Norris (eds), *Amyotrophic Lateral Sclerosis: A Comprehensive Guide to Management*, New York: Demos.

Manton, K. G. and Stallard, E. (1991) 'Cross sectional estimates of active life expectancy for the US elderly and oldest-old populations', *Journal of Gerontology (Social Sciences)* 46: 170–82.

Mitsumoto, H. (1994) 'Classification and clinical features of amyotrophic lateral sclerosis', in H. Mitsumoto and F. H. Norris (eds), *Amyotrophic Lateral Sclerosis: A Comprehensive Guide to Management*, New York: Demos.

Mitsumoto, H. and Norris F. H. (eds) (1994) *Amyotrophic Lateral Sclerosis: A Comprehensive Guide to Management*, New York: Demos.

Mitteness, L. S. and Barker, J. C. (1995) 'Stigmatising a "normal" condition: urinary incontinence in later life', *Medical Anthropology Quarterly* 9: 188–210.

Molgaard, C. A. (ed.) (1993a) *Neuroepidemiology: Theory and Method*, San Diego: Academic Press.

—— (1993b) 'An introduction to neuroepidemiology', in C. A. Molgaard (ed.), *Neuroepidemiology: Theory and Method*, San Diego: Academic Press.

Murphy, R. (1987) *The Body Silent*, London: Phoenix House.

Neilson, S., Robinson, I., and Hunter, M. (1992) 'Longitudinal Gompertzian analysis of ALS mortality in England and Wales, 1963–1990: estimates of susceptibility in the general population', *Mechanisms of Ageing and Development* 64: 201–16.

Neilson, S., Robinson, I., Rose, F. C., and Hunter, M. (1993a) 'Rising mortality from motor neurone disease: an explanation', *Acta Neurologica Scandinavica* 87: 184–91.

Neilson, S., Robinson, I., and Kondo, K. (1993b) 'A new analysis of mortality from MND in Japan 1950–1990: rise and fall in the post war years', *Journal of Neurological Sciences* 117: 46–53.

Neilson, S., Alperovitch, A., and Robinson, I. (1994a) 'Rising ALS mortality in France 1968–1990: increased life expectancy and inter-disease competition as an explanation', *Journal of Neurology* 241: 448–55.

Neilson, S., Robinson, I., and Nymoen, E. (1994b) 'Longitudinal analysis of amyotrophic lateral sclerosis mortality in Norway, 1966–1989: evidence for a susceptible subpopulation', *Journal of the Neurological Sciences* 122: 148–54.

Neilson, S., Gunnarsson, L-G., and Robinson, I. (1994c) 'Rising mortality from motor neurone disease in Sweden, 1961–1990: the relative role of increased population life expectancy and environmental factors', *Acta Neurologica Scandinavica* 90: 150–9.

Neilson, S., Robinson, I., and Rose, F. C. (1996a) 'Mortality from motor neurone disease in Japan, 1950–1990: association with fallout from atmospheric weapons testing', *Journal of the Neurological Sciences* 134: 61–6.

—— (1996b) 'Ecological correlates of motor neuron disease mortality: a hypothesis concerning an epidemiological association with radon gas and gamma exposure', *Journal of Neurology* 243: 329–36.

Neilson, S., Robinson, I., Pedro-Cuesta, J., and Veiga-Cabo, J. (1996c) 'The decline in mortality from motor neurone disease in Spain, 1960–1989: demographic, environmental and competitive influences', *Neuroepidemiology* 15: 180–91.

Nijhof, G. (1995) 'Parkinson's disease as a problem of shame in public appearance', *Sociology of Health and Illness* 17(2): 193–205.

Norris, F. H. (1994) 'Care of the amyotrophic lateral sclerosis patient', in H. Mitsumoto and F. H. Norris (eds), *Amyotrophic Lateral Sclerosis: A Comprehensive Guide to Management*, New York: Demos.

Olivares, L., San Esteban, E., and Alter, M. (1972) 'Mexican "resistance" to amyotrophic lateral sclerosis', *Archives of Neurology* 27: 397–402.

Ory, M. G. and Bond, K. (1989) *Ageing and Healthcare: Social Science and Policy Perspectives*, London: Routledge.

Parks, B. M. (1994) 'Successful home care', in H. Mitsumoto and F. H. Norris (eds), *Amyotrophic Lateral Sclerosis: A Comprehensive Guide to Management*, New York: Demos.

Pearlman, R., Uhlmann, R., and Jecker, N. (1992) 'Spousal understanding of patient quality of life: implications for surrogate decisions', *Journal of Clinical Ethics* 3: 14–20.

Peters, P. K., Swenson, W. M., and Mulder, D. W. (1978) 'Is there a characteristic personality profile in amyotrophic lateral sclerosis?', *Archives of Neurology* 35: 321–2.

Robinson, I. (1988) *Multiple Sclerosis*, London: Routledge.

—— (1990) 'Ethical issues and methodological problems in the conduct of clinical trials in amyotrophic lateral sclerosis', in F. C. Rose (ed.),

Progress in clinical neurological trials. Vol. 1: Amyotrophic Lateral Sclerosis, New York: Demos.

Robinson, I., Hunter, M., and Neilson, S. (1991) 'A new approach to the epidemiology of ALS/MND: problems and possibilities in a national register of patients with ALS/MND', in F. C. Rose (ed.), *New Evidence in MND/ALS Research*, London: Smith-Gordon.

Rosen, D. R., Siddique, T., Patterson, D. *et al.* (1993) 'Mutations in Cu/Zn superoxide dismutase gene are associated with familial amyotrophic lateral sclerosis', *Nature* 362: 59–62.

Rosenberg, L. T. (1993) 'We have a prejudice against ourselves', *Journal of Medicine and Humanities* 14: 5–14.

Rubinstein, R. L. (1990) 'Culture and disorder in the home care experience', in J. F. Gubrium and A. Sankar (eds), *The Home Care Experience*, Newbury Park: Sage.

—— (1995) 'Narratives of elder parental death: a structural and cultural analysis', *Medical Anthropology Quarterly* 9(2): 257–76.

Salander, P., Bergenheim, T., and Henriksson, R. (1996) 'The creation of protection and hope in patients with malignant brain tumours', *Social Science and Medicine* 42(7): 985–96.

Seale, C., Addington-Hall, J., and McCarthy, M. (1997) 'Awareness of dying: prevalence, causes and consequences', *Social Science and Medicine* 454(3): 477–84.

Seckler, A. B., Meier, D. E., Mulvihill, M., and Paris, B. E. (1991) 'Substituted judgement: how accurate are proxy predictions', *Annals of Internal Medicine* 115(2): 949–1054.

Shilling, C. (1993) *The Body and Social Theory*, London: Sage.

Siddique, T., Figlewicz, D. A., Perikvance, M. A. *et al.* (1990) 'Linkage of a gene causing familial amyotrophic lateral sclerosis to chromosome 21 and evidence of genetic locus heterogeneity', *New England Journal of Medicine* 324: 1381–4.

Slater, R. (1995) *The Psychology of Growing Old*, Buckingham: Open University Press.

Sontag, S. (1989) *Illness as Metaphor*, New York: Doubleday.

Swash, M., Swartz, M. S., and Li, T. M. (1989) 'Trends in mortality from motor neuone disease', *Lancet* 335 (letter): 958.

Tandon, R. and Bradley, W. G. (1985) 'Amyotrophic lateral sclerosis: 1. Clinical features, pathology and ethical issues in management', *Annals of Neurology* 18: 271–80.

Tennstadt, S. L. and McKinlay, J. B. (1989) 'Informal care for frail older persons', in M. G. Ory and K. Bond (eds), *Ageing and Healthcare: Social Science and Policy Perspectives*, London: Routledge.

Williams, D. B. and Windebank, A. J. (1991) 'Motor neurone disease (amyotrophic lateral sclerosis)', *Mayo Clinic Proceedings* 66: 54–82.

Williams, G. (1984) 'The genesis of chronic illness: narrative reconstruction', *Sociology of Health and Illness* 6: 175–200.

Williams, R. (1990) *A Protestant Legacy: Attitudes to Death among Older Aberdonians*, Oxford: Clarendon Press.

Index